THE
HEART
OF
CARE

DIGNITY IN ACTION:
A GUIDE TO PERSON-CENTRED
COMPASSIONATE ELDER CARE

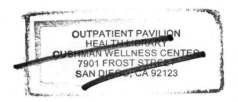
Amanda Waring

Souvenir Press

To my mother and father

Typeset by M Rules
Printed and bound in Great Britain by Page Bros, Norwich

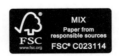

MIX
Paper from
responsible sources
FSC® C023114
FSC
www.fsc.org

FILMS AND PRODUCTS BY AMANDA WARING

What Do You See?

This powerful award-winning short film has been acknowledged as one of the most valuable tools to highlight dignified and compassionate care for the elderly. It is used around the world for inductions into caring careers. The film follows a day in the life of an elderly stroke victim, Elsie, played by Virginia McKenna, who makes a silent, but heartfelt, plea to her carers to "Look closer . . . see . . . me".

Home

Starring Virginia McKenna, *Home* looks at Elsie's arrival in her new care home as she struggles with the transition and mild dementia. This poignant six-minute film helps us understand the emotional journey of an older person during this time.

No Regrets

A daughter visiting her elderly mother in hospital leads to startling revelations about caring, grieving and dying. This sensitive film helps you support and understand the relative's perspective and reminds you that it is never too late to tell someone you love them.

The Big Adventure

Using interviews, poetry and humour, this uplifting and inspiring film examines end of life care and our attitudes towards death to stimulate debate and provide a varied selection of concepts and beliefs. This film is used in many hospices and care settings to challenge and transform care and to embrace the spiritual needs of those who are dying.

THE WHAT DO YOU SEE? TRAINING PACK.

The pack consists of a work book with a DVD of Amanda's films supporting the exercises and a CD Rom containing the handouts required. This motivational pack provides 50 hours' worth of training around dignity.

I AM NEAR YOU CD

This beautiful CD of Amanda's songs and meditations is used in care settings as a comforting presence to those who are maybe dying alone or when care staff and family are unable to be present. Amanda's soothing melodies and healing words help to calm, to uplift and to alleviate a feeling of being alone.

Amanda's award-winning films on dignity and end of life care are available from the online shop on her website www.amandawaring.com

CONTENTS

FOREWORDS

I think it is very important for older people to be listened to and for people to be aware of their thoughts and needs, particularly in a hospital or residential care environment. It is also very important for families to be aware of their older relatives' comforts, mental and physical, as these days the family unit is not as close as it was.

I therefore feel that it is vitally necessary for this book to be written.

Dame Vera Lynn, DBE

The Heart of Care by Amanda Waring makes essential reading for anyone involved in the care and support of older people.

In the 21st century we have become so focused on the technicalities of delivering healthcare that we tend to forget that good quality, compassionate care, which respects the dignity of individuals, has to be at the very centre of the way in which we support our older citizens.

The Heart of Care reminds us that treatment which is devoid of compassion and respect for the individual can have no place in a civilised society.

I recommend this book to all of those who work in the care and support system and to every citizen who intends to get old.

Martin Green
Chief Executive: English Community Care Association
Dignity Commissioner

INTRODUCTION

When my mother, the late great actress Dame Dorothy Tutin, was in hospital awaiting treatment for leukaemia at the age of 70, I witnessed the devastating effect the lack of compassionate and dignified care had on her mind, body and spirit. I witnessed many moments when she and other older patients were treated rudely, with little respect. I remember vividly the lack of communication and interaction between doctors and nurses and my mother during her stay in that first hospital. It was as if she were invisible: human contact was at a bare minimum, with the staff barely making eye contact. This lack of communication was crushing Mama's spirit and she started to withdraw and disengage from life. She said she felt like a caged animal.

That's when my involvement with care of the elderly began, and why I became such a passionate advocate for improving it. I was motivated to educate, inform and inspire those who care for the elderly, and I have since produced films and developed training materials used throughout the country.

In my training sessions and workshops I like to retell the story of American Dr Paul E. Ruskin, MD, who was giving a lecture to graduate nurses on the psychological aspects of ageing. He told them: 'The patient neither speaks nor comprehends the spoken word. Sometimes she babbles incoherently for hours on end. She is disoriented about person, place and time. She does, however, respond to her own name. I have worked with her for the past six months, but she still shows complete disregard for her physical appearance and makes no effort to assist in her own care. She must be fed, bathed and clothed by others. Because she has no teeth, her food must be puréed. Her shirt is usually soiled from almost incessant drooling. She does not walk. Her sleep pattern is erratic. Often she wakes in the middle of the night, and her screaming awakens others. Most of the time she is friendly and happy, but several times a day she gets quite agitated without apparent cause. Then she wails until someone comes to comfort her.

'I asked how the nurses would feel about taking care of such a patient. They used such words as "frustrated", "hopeless", "depressed" and "annoyed". When I said that I enjoyed it and thought they would, too, the class looked at me in disbelief. Then I passed around a picture of the patient: my six-month-old daughter.

'Why is it so much more difficult to care for a 90-year-old than a six-month-old with identical symptoms? A helpless baby may weigh 15 pounds and a helpless adult 100, but the answer goes deeper than this. The infant represents new life, hope and almost infinite potential. The aged patient represents the end of life, with little chance for growth in some aspects. We need to change our perspective. Those who are ending their lives in the helplessness of old age deserve the same care and attention as those who are beginning their lives in the helplessness of infancy.'

As the population ages, more of us will be called upon to care for others. So we must understand the importance of recognising and honouring the intrinsic worth of others, regardless of age or disability. Caring for another human being is sacred work that should have preserving the essence of human dignity at its heart.

This country needs you to be nourished, supported and inspired to give the best care that you can, so let us begin the journey of providing a positive social environment for us all. Let us be mindful that we all have our part to play.

- We will need to cultivate the ability to listen, appreciate, empathise, and celebrate.
- We will need to look at the world from the perspective of an older person.
- We will need to recognise, address and pacify our own fears.
- We will need to examine our own attitudes to and assumptions about older people.
- We will need to develop compassion and deep awareness of the suffering of another, coupled with the desire to relieve it.
- We will need to practise self-care, self-love, and self-responsibility and self-knowledge.
- We will need to keep motivated, to sustain morale and not lose our sense of humour!
- We will need to be brave enough, bold enough, honest enough to ask for help.
- We will need to look at how we can respect wishes, offer choices and give back a sense of control where appropriate.

As a society we will have to accept this challenge, which we can see as a burden or as an opportunity to re-inspire our humanity by sharing one of our greatest attributes: being able to give and receive love.

This book is intended primarily for all professionals – managers, nursing staff, assistants, students – who care for the elderly in hospitals, in care homes, in hospices and in home settings. But everyone who cares for an elderly relative at home, or who has an elder in a hospital or care home, will find much that applies to their needs and challenges too.

This book is intended to be dipped into rather than read straight through, with each chapter refreshing and adding to the principles of delivering the heart of care. Gentle repetition is intended to ensure that these important aspects are understood and put into practice. Even if you have only a few short minutes a day to care for those elders in your charge, I hope you will find new, more effective and more compassionate ways within these pages to connect, communicate and deliver care – as well as ways to care for yourself.

I was delighted to be approached by Souvenir Press to write this book, and welcomed the opportunity to draw inspiration, research and knowledge from the *What Do You See?* training pack which was co-authored by myself and consultant occupational therapist, Rosemary Hurtley.

I approached Rosemary to collaborate on our training pack in 2009 as I recognised a similar passion to improve care of the elderly, and her professional expertise and knowledge was invaluable. I am grateful for the opportunity to share aspects of our work within the body of this book and for the kind permissions granted by Rosemary to also include her important original material from the CD ROM from our training pack including p. 47–56, 92–100 and 128–136.

Permissions have also been granted for including material originally published in Hurtley R, Wenborn J (2005) *The Successful Activity Co-ordinator*, Age Concern England (p. 120–127)
Hurtley R (2010) *Insight into Dementia*, CWR (p. 83–85)

Please note quotation on p. 46–47 is wrongly attributed to Dr Bill Thomas and should be referenced from The Constant Gardner, R Hurtley used in our *What Do You See?* training films (2010).

About the training pack:

> The *What Do You See?* Transforming training pack by Amanda Waring and Rosemary Hurtley:
>
> This learning facilitator pack comprises a trainers manual, DVD with over 20 tracks and unique supporting print-out hand-outs on a CD Rom that are designed to be used in the workplace in flexible 1.5 hour sessions covering many of the issues set out in this book.
>
> It will transform person-centred practice through the use of interactive, immediate and enjoyable group exercises in the workplace that embed behaviours that enable dignity in care.

CHAPTER 1

Dignity at the Heart of Care

Dignified, person-centred care requires getting to the *heart* of things, getting personally involved and motivated rather than staying at the edges or ticking boxes. I guarantee that if your dignity were stripped, or if you witnessed this happen to a loved one, you would march forward with even greater enthusiasm to change society's view and transform the care of our elderly. We need to find that fundamental spark of human kindness and connectedness that provides a foundation of trust and integrity and prevents us from lashing out, disrespecting or dishonouring those in our path.

We must safeguard the emotional wellbeing of those we care for. The victim of emotional abuse can feel bullied, ignored, isolated, discriminated against, devalued and controlled, and we must learn ways to change our behaviour when we are emotionally victimising and dehumanising those we care for.

It is so important to maintain dignity, particularly during intimate caring situations; to have an understanding of frailty and its consequences; and to be aware how much involving older people in their care restores their sense of self-worth. As carers we must understand the difference between ignoring people's needs and providing too much help. We must endeavour to build positive, trusting relationships with those in our care and to adjust the pace of care delivered to suit the individual.

Addressing the a,b,c,d,e of dignity-conserving care – attitudes, behaviour, compassion and communication, dialogue and enablement – shows ways for you to deepen your practice of dignified care.

> 'The duty to uphold, protect and restore the dignity of those who seek care embraces the very essence of medicine and social services' – *A Dignified Revolution (an initiative established in January 2008 to ensure that older people are cared for with dignity and respect)*

Our attitudes towards the elderly

AGEISM IN SOCIETY

Dignity may be promoted or diminished by the attitudes of those caring for older people. Addressing ageism and changing attitudes towards growing older are among the first principles needed when placing dignity at the heart of care. We should not wear age as a burden but a crown.

Let us look at the attitude of ourselves and society to older people. How does this attitude affect what we do and how we respond to older people? We all need to be aware of the power of the media – the profound influence and impact that negative or unbalanced or biased representation can have. I believe that categorising any sector of society prevents a true exploration of all the myriad facets of who we are, and can interfere with our ability to see people as individuals with their own histories, rights and abilities. It is very sad that we are so often unable to acknowledge our true age for fear of negative judgements from others.

We all make judgements, rightly or wrongly, but our inherent prejudices or fears about people can have a damaging effect. When working in care it is really important to address negative attitudes that prevent us from giving respectful care. I have overheard the following judgements from individuals and in the media: 'old people are useless', 'old people are sweet, just like children', 'old people smell', 'old people are ugly and stupid', 'old people are not worth bothering about, they are going to die soon anyway'. Well, we will *all* be old one day (God willing!) and no one wants to be lumped together in such a damning way. These ignorant, thoughtless and cruel judgements destroy our humanity and blind our ability to see the individual inside.

Why in England is being old so often equated to being considered useless? I believe it is because in old age the emphasis can shift from *doing* to *being*. And our civilisation, which is lost in doing, knows nothing of being. But I believe that there is a spirituality and a mystery to allowing ourselves to *be*, an opportunity to discover our values, our essence, what makes us, us.

In Britain the media's obsession with youth does not help the balance of a multi-generational society. All too often older people are ignored, seen but not heard. A balance needs to be restored, before it's too late. Our society is the poorer for this splintering, this disconnection. We need to rediscover community and achieve a balance between independence and interdependence. Our elders are our history keepers, and we can't know where we are going without knowing where we've been.

In British culture the word 'old' has mainly negative associations, but in tribal traditions and other cultures older people are embraced and indeed revered for their knowledge and experience. They are seen as vital and important parts of these communities. In tribal cultural traditions grandparents are seen as figures of great dignity; old age or approaching death providing an opening to the realm of spirit. Old age is seen as a highly valued time for the flowering of consciousness.

We are all worth the same, whatever our age, and the sooner we understand about having respect for ourselves the easier it will be to maintain respect for older people. As we will all eventually approach old age I believe it is essential to instil a positive attitude towards ageing, and cultivate a good degree of resilience too. As Janet Adam Smith said, 'old age is not for sissies!'

THANKING OUR ELDERS

As an antidote to when we judge, ignore, dismiss or are irritated by the elders we care for, I ask attendees in my workshops to try the following exercise.

I begin, 'As a society we are not very good at thanking others, particularly our elders, often leaving it until it's too late. So I would like you to take time now to think of an older person who has made a difference in your life, whether by their love, their humour, a good recipe ... someone who has touched your spirit in a positive way. I would like you to turn to your neighbour and share the memories of the elders that have made a difference to you.'

I watch the audience members get over their shyness at connecting with the strangers sitting beside them, and I give them five minutes to talk. During that time, the energy in the room is transformed into an animated joy of remembrance. Remembering someone they love becomes a point of contact for these attendees; it breaks down the barriers and elicits laughter and indeed some tears too. I always pay particular attention to those who are struggling with their emotions, for I acknowledge the pain of remembrance too, particularly for those who have been recently bereaved. Then I tell them, 'When you remember an older person in this way it becomes easier to view the elders in your care with a deeper vision, seeing them as valued individuals who have been important to others and loved for the difference that they made.'

I then ask the audience to stand and say out loud a big vocal 'Thank you!' I have always been thrilled by everyone's full participation in this, despite our English reserve! The echoes of the heartfelt thanks from so many people ripple round the room, and in the stillness afterwards I sincerely believe that this expression of gratitude has reached their loved ones in some way, even though they may no longer be with us on the earth. After this exercise, I always feel that we are able to work with a deeper conviction and in more meaningful ways. We can offer the elders in our care the same respect we would want for a member of our family.

Try it for yourself. Think of an older person who has made a difference to your life. Perhaps you might consider thanking them in person if possible, or communicating your gratitude in whatever symbolic way would have meaning for you to honour the contribution they made to your life.

THANK YOU, ADIE

One of the reasons I became such a passionate campaigner for older people was because of the influence of my granny Adie Tutin as I grew up. She died when she was 99 years old. She was an amazing woman. She had a very positive attitude to ageing; she used to say, 'Wrinkles are God's way of showing where smiles have been' and 'Older people never lose their beauty, they merely move it from their faces to their hearts'. She was feisty, intelligent, political, compassionate and active. She was – and is, even in death – my inspiration. She followed her values and beliefs diligently but never had a closed mind. She was forever inquisitive about others and their beliefs, and she helped me see the spark in every individual. I will always be grateful for her love and humour and stories.

A PERSONAL REFLECTION ON DIGNITY

As I have described in the introduction, when my mother, the actress Dorothy Tutin, was in hospital being treated for leukaemia at the age of 70, I was appalled at the attitude of the staff to the elderly patients in their care. I stood in my doctor's doorway refusing to budge until he promised me that Mama would be transferred to another hospital. We made the right choice and were rewarded with staff who were friendly, respectful and communicative, and Mama's spirits and health improved. I do not believe that the staff in that first hospital were being deliberately cruel – simply that communication, interaction skills and understanding dignity were not seen as being an important part of helping a patient's recovery. I certainly think they should be. After all, emotional intelligence does not cost anything, and its practice can vastly improve anyone's stay in a hospital or care home.

When Mama died I didn't want to get bitter, I wanted to take action. So I was inspired in 2005 to make my ten-minute film *What Do You See?* I sold my flat in order to make the film as it was too important to me not to be made. It was my first film as a director, and it takes a journey through a day in the life and a life in the day of elderly stroke victim Elsie (played by the wonderful Virginia McKenna). Elsie craves compassion, and understanding of the person she is inside, rather than the useless 'carcass' she may appear on the outside. Elsie makes a silent but heartfelt plea for her carers to 'look closer . . . see *me*'.

My award-winning film has been viewed by millions around the world. It is used to inspire greater compassion and empathy towards those dependent on care, and it illustrates the damaging effect of undignified practice during personal care. It reinforces the importance of treating others as you would wish to be treated no matter what your age, race, colour, creed or disability. I am so grateful that the film continues to gather even greater momentum within hospitals, schools, prisons, universities, care homes, domiciliary agencies and end of life societies, for it means that my mother's death was not in vain.

The film is based around the poem below, written by a nurse, Phyllis McCormack, who was dismayed at the behaviour of her colleagues on their geriatric ward. She originally wrote the poem anonymously in the hospital magazine. I am very grateful to her son Mike for giving me permission to make it into a film.

> *What do you see?*
> What do you see, nurse, what do you see?
> What are you thinking when you look at me?
> A crabbit old woman, not very wise,
> Uncertain of habit, with faraway eyes.
> Who dribbles her food and makes no reply
> When you say in a loud voice, 'I do wish you'd try.'
> Who seems not to notice the things that you do,
> And forever is losing a stocking or shoe.
> Who quite unresisting lets you do as you will;
> With bathing or feeding the long day to fill.

Is that what you're thinking, is that what you see?
Then open your eyes, nurse, you're not looking at me.
I'll tell you who I am, as I sit here so still,
As I move at your bidding, as I eat at your will.
I'm a small child of ten ... with a father and mother,
And brothers and sisters who love one another.
A girl of sixteen with wings on her feet;
Dreaming that soon a true lover she'll meet.
A bride soon at twenty — my heart gives a leap,
Remembering the vows that I promised to keep.
At twenty-five I have young of my own,
Who need me to build a secure and happy home.
A woman of thirty, my young now grow fast,
Bound to each other with ties that should last.
At forty, my young ones have grown up and gone,
But my man stays beside me to see I don't mourn.
At fifty, once more babies play round my knees;
Again we know children, my loved one and me.
Dark days are upon me, my husband is dead ...
I look at the future, I shudder with dread;
For my young are all busy with young of their own,
And I think of the years and the love that I've known.
I am an old woman now, and Nature is cruel,
'Tis her jest to make old age look like a fool.
The body it crumbles, grace and vigour depart,
There now is a stone where I once had a heart.
But inside this old carcass a young girl still dwells,
And now and again my battered heart swells.
I remember the joys, I remember the pain,
And I'm loving and living life over again.
I think of the years ... all too few, gone too fast,
And accept the stark fact that nothing can last.
So open your eyes nurses, open and see ...

Not a crabbit old woman,
Look closer . . . see *me*.

Phyllis McCormack

I believe that the personal story can convey a message far more powerfully than a White Paper or legislation can, for when people's emotions are engaged then change can happen much quicker. We all need a reminder to see people as individuals with their own histories and their own rights, and to remember that good old-fashioned manners can go a long way in helping us to give dignified care.

Dignity and personal care

WASH MY CARES AWAY

I will never forget the time I watched nurses who gossiped to each other while ignoring the elderly woman they were bathing. They treated her as if she were an object and actually hurt her through their lack of attentiveness, moving her body so roughly she cried out. I was only able to witness this event because the nurses had left the door wide open, so that any shred of dignity was lost for the older patient.

I used this as the very first scene of my film *What Do You See?* as a stark reminder for others of the detrimental impact this kind of rude and thoughtless behaviour has. Many carers in the audiences have acknowledged instances when this has happened. It is important to remember that at times there is a fine line between thoughtlessness and abuse.

Bathing another human being is an extremely intimate and private aspect of care. The focus should be on the person being bathed, and on engaging with that individual respectfully in accordance to their wishes and level of comfort. Be mindful of finding out how much they are able to wash themselves; do not automatically take over aspects of personal care because you are rushed for time, as you can rob someone of their dignity and eclipse a person's sense of control.

Don't uncover more than you have to when washing someone. Again, imagine how *you* would feel if you were powerless to wash yourself. Would you feel embarrassed, or that your modesty was being compromised, if a stranger had to wash you? Bear this in mind the next time you are called upon to carry out duties of intimate care; be gentle and kind, for this can feel like a frightening and invasive procedure.

The ritual of bathing can be made into an enjoyable experience by using a favourite bath wash or a softer flannel, adjusting water temperature, and even where appropriate including candlelight or music, and being sensitive to whether the individual wants to talk or not while being washed.

BEHIND CLOSED DOORS

Another important point to be raised when addressing personal care is that all people, whatever their age and physical ability, should be able to choose to use the toilet in private. Some residents in care have been expected to use a commode while staff are in the room! How does this allow for privacy and dignity? We have a duty to challenge this inhumane practice. I hear examples of doors being left ajar or the wishes of those who need escorting to the toilet being ignored so that they are just left to soil themselves. People who need assistance to use the toilet should be able to receive timely and prompt help, with appropriate safety equipment provided, and they should not be left on the commode or bedpan for longer than is necessary.

We must be aware of how our actions cause humiliation to another. I have heard of nurses who, when dealing with overflowing stoma bags, have held their nose and said, 'That stinks, yuk!', humiliating those they are supposed to be caring for. Your response as a carer to odour is vital in maintaining the dignity of the elderly. You can also help maintain an elder's confidentiality by keeping stoma bags hidden out of sight in a locker, for example. The British Geriatrics Society's 'Behind Closed Doors' campaign (www.bgs.org.uk) provides helpful guidelines and standards covering this area of personal care.

COMFORT ROUNDS

After leading dignity workshops at Swindon hospital, I was pleased to hear that they had increased the frequency of their 'comfort rounds' to help with pressure sores, toilet breaks and the provision of drinks. This is an obvious way to enhance dignity in care by increasing nurse/patient communication. Frail patients now have dedicated time and extra contact, and pain can be assessed and monitored more closely. This increase in comfort rounds also reduces the number of call bell summons, which in turn leads to a much calmer environment. I hope this practice will be taken up by all hospitals.

PAIN AND DIGNITY

Pain can strip people of their dignity, keeping them exhausted, vulnerable and disturbed. It is so important that when addressing pain issues you assess the pain from the older person's perspective, which again comes down to monitoring our attitudes and beliefs. I have heard of staff complaining about the elders in their care: 'He needs to man up, he is in there crying like a nine year old' and 'That is just a minor op – he can't be in that much pain.'

Do not let your own uncomfortable reactions to another's pain prevent you from making and recording pain scores on a regular basis. A lot of people internalise their pain, but your friendly approach may help them feel that they are not a bother and to tell you their level of pain. You can then help them manage this. Assess it, believe it, record it, act on it and re-assess. As Margo McCaffery has written: 'Pain is whatever the experiencing person says it is, existing whenever the experiencing person says it does.'

SMALL ACTIONS, BIG DIFFERENCES

Dignity in personal care is demonstrated by ensuring that the spectacles of those in your care are cleaned regularly, that hearing aid settings are corrected where needed, and that all such things are kept within the patient's reach. Fairly obvious actions to take, you would expect, but I am surprised at how often these things can be overlooked. Yet what a positive impact these small adjustments can make. So often it is the small things that can make the biggest difference.

When you brush someone's hair or aid them in brushing their teeth, you can help them restore a sense of control by breaking tasks down into small steps and encouraging them to do as much as they can. As carers we must see our role as someone who assists an individual rather than takes over the task. The latter can foster a feeling of hopelessness and passive acceptance of inevitable decline rather than the possibility of improvement and independence.

Where possible, ensure that personal space is available and accessible when needed to fully respect topics of sensitivity that relate to modesty, gender, culture and religion. Just because you are caring for someone do not assume that you can enter their personal space without permission. Can you make it possible for residents to decide when they want 'quiet time' and when they want to interact?

AN EXERCISE IN DEPENDENCE

Within my workshops I invite carers in pairs to blindfold each other in turn and then take the blindfolded partner's arm as they guide them slowly around the room, where there are obstacles to negotiate. This exercise enables them to feel what it is like to be at the mercy of someone else, to see what level of trust they felt and how vulnerable or supported they felt. After they have put themselves into the shoes of someone who is dependent I ask them to imagine how they would feel if they needed urgent attention and there wasn't anyone to come to their aid. They start to understand the effects of helplessness and long waits for assistance on a dependent person. Imagine if you were even frightened to call staff or if the bell was out of reach?

CHANGING BAD PRACTICE

A friend of mine discovered at her husband's care home that the residents' false teeth were piled in a bowl together with no identification, bleached, then taken back to whomever. My friend complained and the practice was changed, thank goodness.

So take note of any behaviour or practice you have witnessed that takes away dignity, and consider how you could challenge or change a colleague's behaviour. Find out what additional support you may need to do this, or what procedures are in place for raising a concern. Good practice, like bad practice, can spread through a care setting so try to ensure that your knowledge of person-centred care and dignity can be a guiding light for others to follow and learn from. Once a code of behaviour is acknowledged as best practice, then as long as the managers enforce it, it becomes much easier to gently remind others when they are failing the dignity standard expected.

DIGNITY IN COMMUNICATION

It is important to be aware of any barriers that make communication with an older person difficult. Success can be achieved not only by developing the right skills but by modifying behaviour that hinders respectful interaction. Here are some guidelines for dignity in communication.

- It is important *not* to talk about an older person in front of them, or to end up talking for them without asking. Instead, include them as part of the conversation.
- Speak slowly and clearly, allowing enough time and not rushing words.
- Always face an older person at the same level, engaging eye contact and letting them see your mouth.
- Show a nurturing, positive and affirming approach in your tone of voice.
- Don't raise your voice if someone does not understand first time – never shout at an older person or other staff.
- Provide sensitive support, prompting where necessary and allowing people time to express themselves.
- Find out what is important to them, about their life, interests, past achievements, and how they like to be referred to. Use their full title unless given permission to use their first/given name.
- Be honest and preserve trust and integrity, avoiding arguments or confrontation.
- Dignity is dependent not only on *what* is delivered but *how* it is experienced by the person at the receiving end. Speak in a considerate and courteous manner.
- Give an older person as much control as possible over decisions by carefully listening to them and involving them in decision-making about how they like to do things.

- Give encouragement and show interest in what the person is saying.
- Build confidence wherever you can and involve the older person when talking to others.
- Check that the person has understood what is being said before giving more information.
- Ensure hearing aids are worn, and that they have batteries, and that glasses are cleaned regularly.
- Never order, force or coerce someone to participate in an activity, always make every attempt to gain their consent beforehand.
- Before engaging someone in a social activity, make sure they are physically comfortable and observe for signs of pain. Find out how they have slept, enjoyed their meal or whether they need to use the lavatory.
- In social situations link conversations to others; try to encourage links and points of mutual interest for social interaction.

Making mealtimes a dignified experience

Eating and drinking are important daily events that should be enjoyed rather than endured. Giving orders at mealtimes or telling someone off, as in the poem *What do you see?* on page 7, will have a negative impact on a person's self-esteem. Assisting someone to eat a meal requires discretion. Bibs can make people feel that they are being treated like children; large napkins will do just as well. I have been shocked to witness a carer spoon-feeding two individuals at the same time which is of course totally unacceptable.

Think about what can be done to make mealtimes a more dignified and enjoyable activity. Is there anything you can offer others to help them eat independently or more comfortably? Look at specialist equipment such as non–slip mats, large-handled cutlery which is easier to grip, a plate with a lip guard for someone who only has the use of one hand. Find different ways to enable choice and independence during an older person's mealtime, for example offering them jam to spread on their bread or sugar to stir into their tea. If they have a memory problem, remember to prompt at each step – only providing help if necessary by asking them, so as not to take away their dignity or sense of control. Allow them to complete their meal without feeling rushed, for this can force someone to become more dependent and perhaps give up trying altogether. Try to give your complete attention during mealtimes, encourage empathetic listening, and affirm the importance of the right pace of care that promotes independence and choices to maintain a sense of significance and purposefulness.

SOCIABLE MEALTIMES

Carers and elders sharing mealtimes together can be an enriching and social time. You can ask the older person what they particularly enjoy about mealtimes; share favourite recipes together; ask about special memories associated with food, for example Christmas or growing their own vegetables. Consider having themed meals from different countries and be inspired by the music, politics and culture of that region to provide conversation topics. Care homes where staff and residents eat together allow for a family atmosphere, which is a great opportunity to get to know each other in a relaxed way. It also prevents a feeling of isolation, or a them-and-us syndrome developing between staff and residents.

OUT OF REACH

Please don't leave food or drink out of the reach of an older person, which is a common mistake in hospitals and care settings.

Don't clear away the tray untouched without asking if they were physically able to eat their meal without assistance; this is totally unacceptable and unnecessary behaviour. Consider adopting the red tray system, where those who are known to have difficulty eating have food served on a red tray. This provides carers with a visual reminder to assist where necessary.

CREATIVE SOLUTIONS

Making food appetising is particularly important for people who find eating a challenge, have problems chewing or tasting, or who may be feeling unwell or depressed. They need nutritious and attractive meals with right-sized portions presented on a plate. I have met some inspiring chefs who, for people who can only eat puréed foods, use moulds so that instead of an unattractive mush the purée looks like the food it actually is. I found it hard to decipher which was the real cooked English breakfast or its puréed counterpart in one particular care home. Residents there love the new presentation and are eating more and with greater enthusiasm.

'FEED ME' EXERCISE

In my workshops I ask carers to pair up and mix a packet of instant potato mash and hot water in a dish, and to have a glass of water ready as well. They then have to try feeding each other at a slow and a fast pace, with a spoon, in silence. They are to give each other a drink without being asked to do so, and they are not allowed to engage in conversation with the person they are feeding. This is a powerful empathy exercise that brings home the realisation of how institutionalised a person can feel when being treated in this way.

I understand that, with time constraints, not all of my suggestions will be possible all of the time. But think outside the box
when and where you can. Creative solutions can energise
everyone and encourage all to contribute and become re-
enthused about mealtimes. Try to allow older people to be
involved in food preparation where possible, affirming that
their contribution is valuable.

Evolving and maintaining dignity standards

THE NATIONAL DIGNITY COUNCIL

I am so pleased to be on the board of the National Dignity
Council (www.dignityincare.org.uk), an initiative of the Social
Care Institute for Excellence, and the PCOP group (Professionals
Concerned for the Care of Older People). These advisory boards
are committed to shaping care to ensure that dignity and human
rights are at the centre of health and social care. From my meeting the government as a one-woman-band and delivering my
film *What Do You See?* to the then Prime Minister Gordon
Brown and telling them about my dignity campaign and conferences in memory of my mother, I am so delighted to see how
things have grown. The National Dignity Council now has
35,000 'dignity champions' and the website is full of tips, forums
and networking opportunities. As more people grasp the need for
and implementation of dignity the cultural shift will happen, but
we must not take our eye off the ball.

DIGNITY ACTION DAY

A national Dignity Action Day is held by the National
Dignity Council each February. See what you can do for

Dignity Action Day and let me know via the Dignity Council website what success you have had. We can all learn from each other.

EMPATHY AND COMPASSION

The use of empathy and compassion will help us evolve standards of human dignity in care. In 2011 I wrote and recorded my song *We are all the same* for Dignity Action Day as a tool to promote empathy and compassion as vital qualities needed for a more humane society. I am delighted that it is being used at conferences as a rallying cry and call to action, and as a focus for training. My lyrics have been used in poster form as a reminder to put these qualities into practice. You can hear the song on my website www.amandawaring.com

> *We are all the same*
> I am only one
> But still I am one
> I cannot do everything
> But still I can do something
> I will not refuse to do the something
> I can do.
>
> Understand we are all the same
> We all feel love, we all feel pain
> Who are we to judge each other
> Before we judge ourselves?
>
> To respect others, you have to respect yourself
> Respect our elders – we too will be old one day.
> Respect history, diversity, ancestry, respect each other
> No matter what age, race, sex, disability.

Reignite our humanity, be the best that we can be.
Rebuild society, how it was meant to be.

Understand we are all the same
We all feel love, we all feel pain
Who are we to judge each other
Before we judge ourselves?

Create the solution, a dignified revolution,
A world without dignity is not our fate.
We can turn things around
It's never too late.
Drum this to the world. Let these words be heard.
Dignity is not a luxury, dignity is a necessity.
Dignity is not a luxury, dignity is a necessity
For our humanity.

Understand we are all the same
We all feel love, we all feel pain
Who are we to judge each other
Before we judge ourselves?

At the end of a person's life
It will be the love they have received
That they will remember.
Dare to care, dare to connect, dare to care with love.
Know that everything you do, everything you say,
Has an effect on another human being.
Look at how you connect, and how you communicate
Respect.

Understand we are all the same
We all feel love, we all feel pain

Who are we to judge each other
Before we judge ourselves?

I am only one
But still I am one
I cannot do everything
But still I can do something
I will not refuse to do the something
I can do.

ASSESSING DIGNIFIED CARE

Take the dignity standards test below. Answer honestly and mark each challenge out of ten to represent where you think you are as carers, where 1 represents extremely poor practice and 10 represents best practice. Use the scores to plan actions towards further improvements.

- Are we polite and courteous even when under pressure?
  1 2 3 4 5 6 7 8 9 10
- Is our culture about caring for people and supporting them rather than being about 'doing tasks'?   1 2 3 4 5 6 7 8 9 10
- Do our policies and practices emphasise that we should always try to see things from the perspective of the person receiving services?   1 2 3 4 5 6 7 8 9 10
- Do we always ensure that people receiving our services are not left in pain or feeling isolated, depressed or alone?
  1 2 3 4 5 6 7 8 9 10
- Do we have zero tolerance to all forms of abuse?
  1 2 3 4 5 6 7 8 9 10

- Do we listen attentively and encourage people to express their needs and wants?   1 2 3 4 5 6 7 8 9 10
- Do we enable people to maintain the maximum level of independence, choice and control?   1 2 3 4 5 6 7 8 9 10
- Do we always act in accordance with our stated values?
                                                                 1 2 3 4 5 6 7 8 9 10

~

'A test of a people is how it behaves toward the old. It is easy to love children. Even tyrants and dictators make a point of being fond of children. But the affection and care for the old, the incurable, the helpless are the true gold mines of a culture.'

Abraham J. Heschel

CHAPTER 2

Person-Centred Care

'A patient is the most important part of our hospital. He is not an interruption to our work, he is the purpose of it. He is not an outsider in our hospital, he is a part of it. We are not doing him a favour by serving him, he is doing us a favour by giving us an opportunity to do so.'

Bombay Hospital motto

I love the above quote and use it often when I speak at conferences about person-centred care. To move forward in the practice of person-centred care means understanding that those you care for must be placed at the heart of the care you give. Person-centred care has become a bit of a buzzword in the care industry, but my concerns are how often this is genuinely put into practice. There is still too much emphasis on task-orientated care. The emotional support of staff trying their best has to be at the core of services aiming to be person-centred. Leaders of person-centred services never allow the *system* of caring to run them; instead, they remain focused on the importance of people's quality of life, with the emphasis on feelings. As my friend the dementia expert David Sheard states in his series of books 'Feelings Matter Most': 'Person-centred care is about the belief in life that feelings matter most. It is something we "feel" and "are", not just something we "do".'

Person-centred care is crucial to maintaining positive identity. It involves valuing people and those who care for them; treating people as individuals; looking at the world from the perspective of the older person; involving older people in decision making; challenging stereotypes about ageing; and providing a positive social environment.

The value of enabling person-centred care means that there can be greater emotional support and connection with those in your care. It also opens the door to enriched relationships, because to be truly person-centred means getting to know the unique personal history and personality of individuals.

Places of care

To appreciate the value of embedding person-centred care, it is helpful to understand the detrimental effects of being non-person-centred. The following lists are adapted from David Sheard's 'Feelings Matter Most' series of books.

A place that is NOT person centred can be

- a place of boredom or lethargy, where elders are left staring into space
- a place of regimented control, locks, set times and task orientation
- a place where staff are consumed with running the place
- a place that is clinical, smells sterile, lacks atmosphere, lacks vitality
- a place where people are herded into dining rooms to sit through silent mealtimes
- a place where people stay in rather than go out

- a place that is cut off from the outside world
- a place that is soulless and emotionless
- a place that knows nothing about who you were and are

A place that IS person centred will be

- a place that values the individual and their past life
- a place that provides meaningful opportunities to be involved and engaged
- a place that focuses on increasing wellbeing
- a place that promotes the need for people to feel free and not controlled
- a place that feels safe and emotionally secure
- a place where people laugh, express feelings, create and make choices
- a place where individual preferences inform the way of care
- a place where staff receive the same person-centred care as they themselves are expected to give others

Whether you are caring for a loved one from home, or work in hospitals, care homes or in domiciliary care, the principles all apply. I encourage you to examine your place of care and the way you work in context with the negative and positive attributes listed, to see where you fit in this scale, and to take the necessary steps to challenge and then change the culture of care that you find yourself in. List any action points needed for change and find ways to involve older people more in personalising their care. It is an exciting, energising journey when you can work with those in your care as a team, but you may find that you or the organisation need more training in relationship building and specialist communication skills, or that simply being permitted more time to talk with older people about the things that matter to them becomes a more important aspect of care.

To maintain person-centred care means that you should continually examine and adjust your behaviour, attitudes and methods of communication, and drop the 'one size fits all' mentality. The rewards are tremendous.

Knowing me, knowing you

POSITIVE INTERACTION

At the end of my film *What Do You See?* the nurse comes in to draw the curtains without once engaging with or even acknowledging the character of Elsie lying in the bed. The nurse is purely task-orientated, and her behaviour undermines Elsie's sense of significance as a valued human being. I ask those in my workshops to role play this scene, showing how this task can be done differently, involving the older person respectfully and making them feel that they matter.

Take every opportunity to engage with those you care for, especially during necessary tasks. This will prevent the older person feeling as if they are just a body to be done unto. Do not dress someone, brush their hair or bathe them in silence. Be confident enough and interested enough to share conversation, sing together even, share jokes and memories. Sharing and even preparing a meal together provides further opportunities for engagement. You can help mealtimes become a more person-centred experience when there is greater focus on the atmosphere during a meal. Consider music, how you place each person at the table, lighting, fresh air. Match portion size to each person's need, use finger foods and foods from the past to stimulate memories. Make the personal personal! Try to support those in your care to feel confident enough to express what they really want, and to see a connection between your learning and their living.

THE ELEMENT OF TRUST

Understand that we all wear many masks in our interaction with people. So it may take some time for us as individuals to feel safe enough with another person to let our masks slip. I always feel it is important to share aspects of your own life with those you care for; in this way you are bringing the outside world in to the world of older people. It is an interesting exercise to consider how you present yourself to others, and how much this is really a reflection of the person you are inside. Certain difficult behaviour in others is there to express a need rather than that person just being awkward for the sake of it, so I invite you to see beyond the masks of yourself and those you care for to reveal the true person inside through gentle coaxing and patience. Nothing needs to be rushed. The element of trust in person-centred care is vital.

Offering person-centred care requires you to be on a continuous journey of discovery. Keep learning, observing and listening, placing those you care for at the heart of what you do. Endeavour to find out what they most enjoy about life, what are their hopes and fears, what would they like people to know about them and how they would like to leave their mark before the end of their life. You must always respect the privacy of what is shared with you in confidence, for you will learn so much more when you are worthy of trust.

SHARING REMINISCENCES

It is necessary to understand the life experience of an older person to support their individuality. Such things as photographs, objects or ornaments are important visual and tactile symbols of someone's significant memories and achievements, especially for people with dementia. These 'memory joggers' can assist their recall and sense of individuality. Encourage the placing and use of these mementoes with those in your care, seeking assistance from relatives if necessary.

Spend time to explore and reminisce, and share your stories too. Promoting person-centred care means that you get personally involved. Think of a memory from your own past. What object would you use to represent this? How might this help to restore and share a memory with someone else? Share objects with those in your care, share your world and enjoy theirs. When I give talks I often hand out lavender from my garden to those present. People are often quite surprised by this interaction. It is a small gesture, but it is appreciated. Consider making this something you can do on a regular basis.

CHAPTERS OF MY LIFE

I really enjoy doing this David Sheard exercise when I work with relatives, staff and residents in care homes. It is simple but fun, and enables a greater personal connection and understanding of each other's lives. I ask them to imagine that a book publisher wants to offer each of them a one million pound advance for their autobiography. All he requires is the title of the book and five chapter headings. I then give them five minutes to think about this before sharing their 'books'. This is such a revealing exercise. It is life stories in miniature, and can open up discussion around the themes and the titles. I always encourage the possibility of them feeling inspired to actually write the book, or perhaps make a book cover that can be shared by all.

Try this, for it has an immediate impact. It enables carers and elders to share their autobiographies through these teaser titles, and encourages expansion.

QUESTIONS TO ASK YOURSELF

Vulnerable older people can feel crushed and withdraw into passivity if attitudes around them are controlling and behaviour towards them is task-orientated. So how can you become more person-centred when caring for another? Think about the following questions: What time is built into the care hours to address this important aspect? How can you demonstrate good listening and communication skills to involve and include older people more in everyday life?

I stress in my talks that everyone has a set of habits, rituals and different ways they like to do things whatever age they are. By identifying your own preferences, you can appreciate more the importance of supporting others to have their needs catered for. You will need to try to identify preferences around personal care through asking relatives or friends for those with communication or memory problems. Answers to these questions are important and will help you deliver true person-centred care. Below is a checklist of questions to find answers to where possible for those you care for:

- What are their favourite drinks (hot, cold, alcoholic)? How do they like their drinks served?
- What are their favourite foods? Which foods do they dislike? What are their preferred times of eating? Do they require special cutlery?
- Which items of clothing do they prefer to wear? What accessories do they normally wear?
- Do they require any rituals around bedtime to assist sleep? Which nightwear, bedclothes, number of pillows, lighting and ventilation do they prefer? How do they like to wake up in the morning?

- What is their preferred time and method for bathing? Do they have special items that should be used?
- Do you know what they prefer to use for hair care, skin care, makeup, nail care, aftershave or perfume? What about hairdressing needs and style preferences?
- What can they do for themselves, and what do they need help with?
- What do they enjoy doing during the day? Where do they like to sit? Do they have any particular routines they like to follow? Which conversation topics do they enjoy?
- What do you know about their anxieties or fears? What things make them feel upset or angry? Can you tell when they are upset? How can you tell when they are contented?
- Do they have any significant close relationships?

Celebrating difference

MAKE AN EFFORT

It often requires more effort if people who are either the givers or the recipients of care come from a different background, ethnicity or culture, so it is important to be aware of the guidelines below.

- Examine your own prejudices.
- Be aware of the language that you are using.
- Learn something about the ways in which respect is shown in different cultures.
- Be aware of the meaning of different gestures, the use of personal space and touch, etc.
- Try to learn greetings in different languages, particularly if

you have a high ratio of people who do not speak English.

- Try to involve volunteers who can interpret instructions for people for whom English is a second language.
- Encourage individuals from different ethnic groups to use crafts, skills and knowledge to portray their own culture. For example, Chinese calligraphy, while being a written language, can also make a framed picture. Some individuals may remember traditional recipes to share.
- Be aware of different ethnic foods and dress. Bring in some examples and have a celebration day of 'difference'.

(Adapted from Network Publishing, 2006)

FURTHER RESEARCH

To deepen your person-centred approach to those from different backgrounds, consider the following points and discover as much as you can to assist your understanding. Be aware of non-verbal and verbal means of communication.

- How long has the older person lived here? What is the history of their migration, customs and traditions, social groups?
- How much do you know about their family unit – its cohesiveness, size, beliefs, roles, attitudes to care?
- What is their perception of age? What are their social attitudes to others, especially in regard to stereotyping and myths?
- What is their level of English usage? Remember that some people in later stages of dementia slip into their mother tongue.
- What are their attitudes to gender, in particular towards segregation in relation to eating, cooking and religious activity?

- What are their customs and traditions associated with food and diet?
- What are their religious practices, beliefs and values? Do they celebrate festivals and religious traditions, and if so what are the significant dates?
- How do they like to dress? Are there areas of potential offence?
- What are their culture's attitudes to death and dying? Are there special beliefs, rituals and customs around the subject?
- What are their attitudes towards intimate personal care?

(Adapted from the National Association for Providers of Activities for Older People, NAPA, 2002)

Person-centred care and dementia

People living with a dementia come to rely less on thinking and more on feeling. Providing emotional care is therefore vital and requires giving of yourself emotionally to reach out to, connect with and support those in your care. When people are working in this way they need to be supported themselves, through informal daily measures such as debriefing, chatting, and opportunities to reflect at the end of the day's caring. More formal approaches, through reflective supervision, group support sessions, learning opportunities to explore emotions at work, are invaluable. External counselling avenues are also helpful.

Being emotionally engaged with those in your care can leave you feeling drained, exhausted and empty, so it is important that you as a carer find ways to recharge your batteries. The chapter 'When the going gets tough' provides insights, tools and exercises to help prevent burnout.

FOREWARNED IS FOREARMED

David Sheard's work highlights areas where person-centred care has the potential to create misunderstandings or even conflict with families not versed in this approach, because person-centred care works on respecting the person with dementia as they are now, not how they once were.

'Dignity and choice has to be focused on who the person with dementia is now, taking precedence over who the person was,' he writes. 'In practice this can mean supporting someone in a different reality. The person may be wearing clothes differently, making food choices differently, occupying themselves differently, seeking new relationships differently from the way they have done in the past. Person-centred care accepts that forcing a past reality and using logic and reason will not work.'

Families who see it as their role to maintain a person's past wishes can strongly resist the practices of person-centred care, so skilful negotiation and communication to enable working in partnership with families may be required. Relatives' input is vital, so it is important to reach a clearly defined consensus.

'Remember the days of old, consider the years of many generations: ask thy father, and he will shew thee; thy elders, and they will tell thee.'

The Bible

CHAPTER 3

From Home or Hospital
to Care Home

This chapter explores the impact of moving into a care home, and how families and carers can aid this transition. We must give time, patience, compassion, understanding and emotional support to ease the transition, for moving into a care home is a major life event and involves massive upheaval whatever the circumstances.

The impact of transition

DEVASTATION OR REGENERATION?

The impact of change on each person will vary. Change can affect people's physical, mental, emotional and social equilibrium. People manage transitions differently through life. Some people cope well with big events and others can be demolished by small ones. Moving into a care setting means not only the act of settling in but also fitting in with others along the way.

Some people may even have to move on again if their care needs change or if circumstances require relocation. Moving into a care home is often done at a time of crisis, following an illness, hospitalisation, or the death of a spouse or carer, so there are already strong emotional challenges present.

A residential setting has the potential to be a lifesaver for someone who is lonely, isolated and disconnected from people as their friends and family are no longer around. But our individual nature will determine our attitude to such a move. We must understand the anxieties of someone who is unsure whether they are moving into a community of emotional support or whether they will be spending the rest of their days in an institutionalised environment.

LOSING WHAT YOU KNOW

Even though many older people actively and happily make the choice to move into a care home, it can feel like a bereavement as it is about the multiple loss of home, possessions, independence and a sense of control over one's life. However attractive, homely or comfortable a care home might be, it does not compensate for the initial trauma of the loss of the familiar.

PUT YOURSELF IN THEIR SHOES

To enable others to identify with an older person moving into a care home, during my talks I ask care staff to really think of the impact it would have on their own lives if they had to move into a care home *today*.

How would it feel to be taken away from your husband or wife, your children, your home? How would it feel to lose your interaction with street life, village life, community and friends? To lose all those small social interactions that made up your day – chatting with the neighbours, shopkeepers and postman, seeing the local kids grow up? How would it feel knowing that you would not be sleeping in your bed again, or smelling the flowers in your garden, or touching your banister as you climb up the stairs? The smells, the touch, the sights, the sounds – all our senses are involved in the way we frame our world. The context of who you are and what you know . . . those threads would feel as though they were breaking as you lost your home, full of memories and lifelong treasured possessions.

In 2009 I made my short film *Home*, which again stars Virginia McKenna as Elsie, the character she played in my 2005 film *What Do You See? Home* highlights the sense of displacement that can be felt when moving into a care home, especially for someone who has dementia, and emphasises the need to assist transitions sensitively and positively. I am so pleased this film has been used productively in training programmes around the world to open carers' eyes to the experience of an older person entering a care home. The film was always intended to support the emotions of transitions rather than condemn the placing of an older person in a care home, particularly as this may be the best solution for those who need it.

Home
They took me to this house, this very nice house,
With nice front steps and a nice big hall.
'This is were you live now,
Mummy,'
They told me.
But it isn't my house at all.

They took me round the garden, this nice big garden,
With nice bright borders and a high brick wall.
'This is where you walk now,
Mummy,'
They told me.
But it isn't my garden at all.

They took me to a bedroom, this nice big bedroom,
With a nice colour telly, and prints on the wall.
'This is where you sleep now,
Mummy,'
They told me.
But it isn't my bedroom at all.

They took me to a lounge, this nice sunny lounge,
Full of old dears, who said nothing at all.
'These are your friends now,
Mummy,'
They told me.
But they're not *my* friends at all.

They got into their car, their nice big car,
And they waved goodbye just before nightfall.
'This is your life now,
Betty,'
I murmured.
But it isn't my life at all.

Christopher Matthew, Now We Are 60
(and a Bit), *Hodder & Stoughton, London, 2003*

Coping with change

ASSIST ME

Think what it might be like to be the character in the poem above, who perhaps has mild dementia and has been in hospital before moving into a care home without adequate preparation. Or perhaps she moves in knowing it is for the convenience of her relatives, or so as not to be a burden – all complex emotive scenarios. She is disorientated and constantly searching for something familiar and meaningful to find security in life. Think what it might be like to move into a new environment where there is no one you know, and where the routines and layout are so different from those you are familiar with.

In my workshops I ask carers again to put themselves in the shoes of an older person and provide answers to some of the following questions, adapted from the website www.myhome-lifemovement.com.

- What would you like staff to know about you to help you settle in?
- What kind of support might you need to come to terms with the loss of your home, your health, your loved one/s?
- What could the home do to make you feel welcome, cared for and valued?
- What would be your main fears about going into a care home, and what might help alleviate these fears?
- What possessions would you hope to bring with you to the home?
- How could you be helped to remain linked to the past, to old friends, hobbies and places?
- What things in life are most important to you?
- What would help you feel positive about the future?

THE NEW ARRIVAL

If I moved into a care home I would want the care staff to assist me in a new way of living, to see *me*, to understand *me*, to involve *me* in creating this new community I found myself in. Especially in those first days and nights, when my feelings would be running high and my emotions near the surface. I would want to feel that my needs would be listened to. I would want to be able to build up a trusting relationship with the staff.

So how can we help residents in our care to adjust to this transition, and provide assistance with both the acceptance of and adaptation to this new set of circumstances? The checklist below, adapted from *Find the Right Care Home* by Rosemary Hurtley and Julia Burton Jones (Age UK, 2008), suggests ways to help. You may wish to add ideas of your own.

- Think about different ways of involving relatives in the important things which might help a person at this time of change and uncertainty – relatives can hold the thread of continuity, particularly for people with dementia.
- Help residents become familiar with their new environment and routines by explaining things, affirming, reminding and encouraging, and involving relatives and friends where possible during the settling-in period.
- Encourage residents to keep up their relationships with friends, members of their family and organisations of significance to them by helping, if possible, with correspondence, emails, Skype etc.
- Share the emotional aspects of the move with residents, helping them to restore a sense of balance and equilibrium.

- Help them to maintain a sense of self and of control, such as in personalising rooms and asking relatives to pass important personal information on if residents cannot speak for themselves.
- Encourage other staff members to find out about individual life stories, which can help to put the present into perspective.
- Involve new residents and/or their relatives in the community life of the home, for example by suggesting different activities, roles and activity groups they might enjoy.
- Encourage decision-making in aspects of the life of the home and ideas for improvements in the settling-in process.
- Introduce residents to the outdoors and to different aspects of the home early in their stay so that they can familiarise themselves with and feel confident in their surroundings.
- Assess how much support will be needed to help participate in social activities.
- Create a 'neighbourhood' of friends, seeking out kindred spirits and encouraging links across and between staff, residents and relatives both formally and informally.
- Provide information and learning opportunities for relatives through groups and seminars.
- Ensure that new residents are introduced to night staff to reassure them that they won't be forgotten and they won't feel as if strangers are assisting them at night.

So what does it mean for a care home when a new resident arrives? It should be about welcoming a new member of the community, and the family, and addressing the change in balance of adding a new personality to the mix. Inviting a prospective resident and family to join for a meal or even a trial weekend is a good idea.

Of course, other residents can help new residents settle in. In a care home in Diss they have one or two residents who like to meet and greet new arrivals. These residents can also show the new ones that life is not over just because they are in a residential home! Residents and relatives from a care home in Sheffield worked together to produce a welcome booklet, including their personal stories of moving into the home, which has been a good support.

Don't leave the family out

INVOLVING FAMILIES

Both my grandmothers, who lived to be 99 and 101 years old, made their own decisions about entering a care home, preferring that option to living with family members because they felt they would have more independence and the surety of any medical needs being met on the premises. My grandmothers visited many care homes before making their final – happy – decisions. Their care homes provided a caring, nurturing, 'other family' environment for which I was so grateful. It was always a joy to visit – and I still keep in touch with the managers after twenty years!

Supporting and encouraging relatives to continue to be involved in the care of their loved one is crucial. A few phone calls by the care staff to the relatives in the first week to keep them updated on how the resident is settling in can make a world of difference. Understand that the relatives will be having complex emotions around this change, ranging from guilt and shame to relief and joy.

Settling in to a care home involves the relatives' important input and knowledge of their loved one. Below is a list of ways to encourage the involvement of relatives during the transition period and beyond.

- Involve relatives in activities, personal care and laundry, room layout, and linking care to former lifestyle, helping residents to retain their identity and sense of control.
- Relatives can help to ensure that links with former life are maintained, through writing letters, emails etc.
- Encourage relatives to bring in favourite foods, games, music etc.
- Encourage relatives to sit and talk with their loved one as often as they can, sharing the emotional aspects of the move.
- Suggest that relatives use favourite activities, photos and scrapbooks as a constant reminder of meaning in life and provide ideas to staff about activities their relative might enjoy.
- Relatives can help staff to understand why their relative behaves or responds in certain ways.
- Encourage relatives to monitor the resident's wellbeing, ensuring lifestyle and clothing, for instance, are consistent.
- Relatives can negotiate and mediate in a range of decisions, from meals to foot care, which are important to the residents.
- Encourage relatives to take their family member outside and enjoy the garden together, to help them get to know the spaces around them early in their stay.

CHECKLIST TO HAND TO FAMILY MEMBERS

This list below might be helpful to give to relatives, to help them think about the aspects of living that can make all the difference to their loved one in care. If staff have enough knowledge they can be more sensitive to important things such as little habits, ways a person likes things to be done, where they need support. Spend some time looking through this list together and discuss why these details may be important, particularly for those with memory difficulties.

How a person likes to be addressed (first/given name, Mr, Dr, Mrs, Ms etc):

Place of birth:

Significant or special places:

Family structure:

Education (favourite school subjects, level reached):

Important life events (births, deaths, marriages, divorce):

Occupation (significant experience in working life, awards etc):

Personality type (for instance, open and chatty or quiet and reserved; what motivates and influences mood):

Social background:

Important values and cultural/religious beliefs:

Pets:

Likes/dislikes (food, pastimes, entertainment, music, TV, radio):

Favourite activities and hobbies:

Skills and talents:

Fears/anxieties:

For those with communication or memory problems, ask about such things as favourite drinks and food, clothing, bedding and bedtime rituals, bathing routines, appearance preferences, companionship likes and dislikes (for example, male or female company, pets, comforters), levels of ability, 'touch' likes and dislikes, names of family and friends, significant visitors and preferred staff, favourite activities and interests, some idea about former significant carer relationships.

(Adapted from Find the Right Care Home *by Rosemary Hurtley and Julia Burton Jones, Age Concern, 2008.)*

~

'Home is where the heart is.'
Traditional

CHAPTER 4

Creating a Thriving Care Home

'You don't stop doing things because you grow old. You grow old because you stop doing things.'

Dame Thora Hird

This chapter looks at enabling meaningful living for elders living in care settings. The social environment should recognise that all human life is grounded in relationships and that older people deserve an enriched social environment which both compensates for their impairments and fosters opportunities for personal growth. An older person who is vulnerable or frail might have few expectations, their self-belief and sense of identity is already diminished. It is likely that they will withdraw, accepting whatever comes their way, passively accepting the status quo. That is when exasperation, boredom and tiredness can take over.

THE CONSTANT GARDENER

The idea of a care home being like a garden, with the leader as a constant gardener, is a concept promulgated by the Eden

Alternative, an organisation dedicated to improving the experience of elders in care homes (www.eden-alternative.co.uk). Dr Bill Thomas, the founder of the Eden Alternative, has stated: 'Care settings are complex, changing communities, dependent on good leadership that involves and supports staff, residents and relatives. A good manager is like a constant gardener, watering, feeding, tending, pruning, guiding, learning – creating a place that feels good to live in, good to work in and good to visit.

'Each plant in this garden is unique, despite some similar groupings, offering a rich, vibrant environment filled with diversity, relating together to make the garden a community. This garden needs its own supply of sunlight, water and nourishment for the soil. In Eden terms, the sunlight is the quality of loving companionship and reciprocity providing the warm conditions for growth in the soil.

'Plants also need the water of relationships for the soil, representing spontaneity and "unexpected happenings". The food in the soil nourishes and enables growth, representing an understanding of each individual and what is meaningful for them, matching their abilities to varied tasks and roles within this community.

'The air around the plants represents a gentle encouragement of movement and a quality of life enabled by Life Assistants together with smart attention to health needs to prevent blockages in the system and allow flow. This helps to create the human habitat necessary to prevent loneliness, helplessness and boredom and highlights the principles of closeness, connection, human growth, leadership and shared experiential learning.'

Those of us who work in care homes are 'world makers'. We have the power to make a world of difference by the way we do things and the efforts we make to create a sense of continuous community building. This is achieved by stimulating positive relationships across and between residents, staff and relatives and it is everybody's business to be part of this.

HOW DOES MY GARDEN GROW?

If you are working in a care home setting I encourage you to explore this exercise, which I use in my own workshops.

Ask the group to think about the type of garden your home represents and what part they each play in this garden. Try to involve staff, residents and visitors, and find out about their skills and abilities. What can they bring to the garden? Do they have a hidden talent? Do they play an instrument, cook, or have a skill in some particular craft? Perhaps someone has recently been somewhere interesting, or has a significant event or hobby that they can share. Try to involve and motivate as many people to contribute as possible. *Everyone* can contribute something!

THREE TYPES OF COMMUNITY

Let's explore further the strengths and weaknesses of your care community. Look at the three types of community listed below. Which community does your care setting represent? Use this list to compare and adjust areas where necessary to improve the experience of the residents in your community, and to make your care setting a flourishing place of growth and learning.

A controlled or institutionalised care setting is one where
- there is a sterile environment with little activity or social interaction and no involvement with the community

- elders feel isolated, bored and disengaged, and suffer a loss of independence and confidence
- there is very little access to the outdoors

A 'make-do' care setting is one where
- activity is provided, but with a 'one size fits all' mentality; elders have very little involvement in the choice of what is on offer and people with dementia cannot engage in the activities
- elders feel helpless and passive
- outdoor access is limited and there is only a little contact with the community
- no new learning opportunities or roles are provided
- little training is provided for activity co-ordinators, who are seen as a soft option and not a vital element

A thriving care setting is one where
- activity, both planned and spontaneous, is personal and relevant and includes those with dementia, where personal growth and development are encouraged
- enthusiastic management and leadership are seen as essential, and roles are actively developed
- there is easy access to the outdoors, with good use of the surrounding environment and a balance between safety and freedom
- active decision-making involves residents and relatives as well as staff

YOUR IDEAL CARE HOME

After you have examined your care home community, take ten minutes to think about your own ideal care home. Write down the things you would want; if we are to transform our future care it starts with small steps that we can highlight now. Many who have done this exercise have thought more deeply about the atmosphere and odour in their environment and have taken creative, enjoyable steps to de-sterilise their care home community, transforming the more institutional aspects into homely ones. Some bake fresh bread in the home, or use aromatherapy diffusers, others have music played in the bathrooms. I have so enjoyed the range of individual preferences expressed in this exercise, down to the smell of roasting coffee beans, pets, a herb garden, opportunities to help create meals, music lessons, waterbeds, a gym, salsa nights, lilies in the rooms, large windows, thick rugs, fairy lights, film clubs, wine tastings . . .

Future generations who enter into care will have vastly different tastes in leisure and hobby pursuits to previous generations. Our perception of an 'old person' will change quite dramatically over the next decades, when more vocal generations will not be so stoically passive in their care. The TV personality Janet Street Porter once said that she wanted a care home with a shopping mall. For many 'baby boomers' this is an important leisure activity.

The following list is a useful guide to what has been expressed as a measure of a good care home for the current generation of elders. It is based on the 360 Standard Framework, a standard of excellence in relationship-activated, person-centred care advocated by the 360 Foundation, founded by Pat Duff and Rosemary Hurtley (www.360fwd.com).

Measures that residents use to judge their experience of a good care home
- Receiving person-centred care to acceptable standards
- Having opportunities to occupy my time meaningfully
- Being enabled to influence my food and drink
- Being enabled to meet my spiritual and religious needs
- Being enabled to resolve my concerns and complaints

Measures that relatives use to judge their experience of a good care home

- Welcoming ambience of the home
- Effective communication among residents, staff and managers, and relatives – the relationship triangle
- Being fully informed of events affecting residents' wellbeing (where the resident wishes this)
- Being able to raise concerns and complaints on behalf of a resident without fear of retaliation
- Being welcomed to continue a caring role, being involved in decisions and in the community life of the home

Measures that staff use to judge their experience of being enabled to deliver good care

- Whether they find the work fulfilling
- Having time to deliver good care
- Being equipped to do the job properly
- Feeling valued as a member of staff

ENGAGING THE SENSES IN A CARE HOME

All of our senses are engaged when we enter any environment, but many of us have a preferred, or dominant, sense: seeing, hearing, smelling, touching or tasting. I ask my workshop participants if they know what their dominant sense is, and why? I then ask them to imagine that they were unable to use that sense to relate to the world around them. How would that make them feel?

Then I ask them to take away another sense, and one more. This helps participants understand the impact on older people when their senses may be diminished. Having a range of sensory activities adapted to the abilities and needs of the residents, particularly those with dementia, where you can help them continue to enjoy both the new and the familiar, is really important. Involving everyone – staff, residents and relatives – to come up with ideas together can be stimulating and fun. It can expand the way we all individually respond to our environment, making it a richer and more varied experience.

The following lists of things to enjoy, choose or create using each of the senses give some pointers for you to expand upon.

Seeing

Large pictures or colour prints, including conversation pieces (landscapes, daily life genre, pictures that tell a story)

Retro themed scenes or murals in public areas such as corridors

Art appreciation classes, perhaps engaging local colleges of art

Photography classes

Various art techniques (see list on pages 94–96)

Poetry or prompt words to encourage reminiscing

Outdoor colours, shapes, reflections

Reminiscence/comfort treasure boxes

Hearing

Music to stimulate memory, to enjoy and relax to, or to energise

Singalongs

Poetry recitals

Readings of favourite texts

Garden and everyday sound recordings

Sound effects

Sound quiz

Smelling

Different everyday objects in jars to trigger memories and discussion: herbs, scented plants

Perfumes, talcum powder, bath oils

Cooking smells

Household/DIY smells such as furniture polish, mothballs, washing soaps, sawdust

Old remedies such as camphorated oil, cod liver oil, Vic

Tasting

Different foods, including sweets, savouries, jams, chutneys

Tastes from the past

Different teas, coffees, other drinks both hot and cold

Touching

Simulate daily experiences from the past: feet in water or sand, countryside objects, to trigger reminiscences and shared memories

Sensory blankets, cushions, aprons; objects with tactile qualities of rough/smooth, hot/cold; beads, buttons

Vibrating or moving sensations; massage- or touch-based therapies

Water-based activities

Finding objects in a bowl of rice or lentils

Feely bags

Gardens: plants that are smooth, rough, spiky, soft to touch

Comfort treasure boxes of personal artefacts

PURPOSEFUL MOVEMENT

It is also important to encourage purposeful movement, such as cleaning, dusting, sorting, washing. Indoor activities could include dancing, rocking, exercising to music; outdoor activities could include walking, growing vegetables and flowers, general gardening tasks, hanging out washing. Those who are able could pursue throwing and catching games.

A HOME TO ENJOY

Creating a home to enjoy also means addressing and providing positive solutions to orientation; choice and decision making; personalised space; spirituality; meeting and greeting others; different roles; everyday activities.

The following is a useful checklist to enhance the enjoyment of those you care for.

Orientation: ensure that clear signs act as support and visual invitations at eye level. These can take a number of forms and can supplement words with pictures, images or recognisable symbols. Objects can be very useful for assisting way-finding and help orientation as major 'landmarks'.

Choice/decision making: to encourage these, create spaces where people can relax away from constant noise, bright lights or being watched; where they can just 'be', away from activity places.

Personalised spaces: encourage the expression of individual likes and dislikes using pictures, furnishings and objects of significance.

Spirituality: a quiet corner that may be designed for prayer or worship would support expression of individual cultural and spiritual identity.

Meeting and greeting others: provide opportunities for people to get to know each other through activities such as board games, photographs or objects for discussion, and music (at appropriate times, for appropriate people).

Different roles: use staff knowledge of individual biographies to create opportunities for relationships to be developed and encounters with staff to be meaningful. Enough time and space should be available to enable meaningful social interactions. This involves making 'events' out of different everyday activities as opportunities for communication, celebration, choice, decision-making and shared expression.

Everyday activities: in addition to other types of occupational activity, attention should be paid to the experiences of waking up, dressing, bathing, mealtimes and retiring to bed. Transform the ordinary into the extraordinary!

WISHES FOR A LOVED ONE

The following list is collated from thoughts of relatives of those with dementia on aspects of what they consider to be important in their loved one's care home. Consider your own care setting and ask the relatives and residents where you are getting it right and what can be improved upon. Staff will have their own ideas too; keep the flow of ever-changing ideas, and accept and adapt to realistic criticisms. The confidence this will give to relatives and residents will be of great value.

- There is an established central point or 'heart' of the home where residents can find help, information and company. This is often the kitchen or sitting room in a domestic home.
- Appropriate environmental cues are provided to orientate residents with sensory and/or cognitive impairment, for example large, clear clocks, calendars, text and pictorial signs, colour coding.
- Appropriate equipment and adaptations are provided to enable residents to move around the home freely, such as walking aids, ramps, rails and banisters. This helps to prevent isolation and unnecessary dependence.

- The environment contains a variety of interesting items to stimulate all the senses and to orientate residents. This is particularly important for people with cognitive impairment. Suitable items include: fish tanks, rummage baskets, reminiscence objects such as old work tools. These need to be readily accessible for residents and staff to use. Corridors should be broken up with seating or 'landmarks', clocks, plants, windows, pictures, maps.
- There is a good range of available music, books and video films which reflects residents' interests and preferences, which is being selected, used and changed appropriately throughout the day.
- Radio and television use is appropriate to the wishes and interests of residents, who are consulted on their preferences. Programmes and channels are checked on a regular basis to ensure active choices and selections are made.
- There is easily distinguishable communal and activity space, for example: relaxing quieter areas, dining room, TV room, social lounge, kitchenette.
- A range of appropriate seating is provided throughout, including seats of various heights, colours, textures; arranged to encourage social interaction or provide an interesting view, for example into the community or garden.
- Lighting levels are bright and where possible natural. Glare is reduced wherever possible to prevent disorientation and/or perceptual problems occurring.
- Residents can be seen moving about freely and safely, participating in daily life and interacting with objects around them.
- Residents can be seen making full use of the environmental facilities to promote conversation and

enjoyment, eg looking out of the window and chatting about the view, selecting and playing music.

- There is no unnecessary noise, particularly institutional noise such as repeated unattended bells.
- There is a secure and safe garden, with comfortable seating, appropriate ramps, rails and signage, and freely accessible to residents: the door is unlocked. Residents can be seen moving around freely.
- Residents' individual accommodation is personalised with familiar pictures and objects that have emotional appeal, along with books, newspapers etc. Each room looks different from the next.
- Facilities are provided for visiting children, for example a children's corner with bean bags, books and toys.
- There is NO evidence of institutional features, for example: unattended linen, dining or tea trolleys, wheelchairs; staff notice boards in communal areas, or notices for residents produced in illegible format or placed too high to be read.

QUALITY CARE AT NIGHT

Our ability to build a relationship with an elder is greatly enhanced when there is as much unbroken sleep as possible. However, night time can be a very difficult time for residents. For some, used to the company of a husband or wife at night, the isolation can be distressing. So, when working as night staff, welcome these residents to come and join you. These quiet periods often allow staff to get to know residents better, sitting quietly together on a one to one basis, being able to listen to any concerns and explore their wants and needs. Some night-time staff have created individual care plans for residents at night which are hugely effective at communicating the night-time needs of residents.

Although noise and light are sometimes unavoidable, keep assessing how they may be affecting residents' sleep. Between the TV and the dishwasher, buzzers, pagers and staff talking, the noise at night can be overwhelming. Minimise noise where possible and install movement-sensitive lighting so the light will dim or go out once the person has moved on.

Some relatives worry about their loved one's sleep patterns and care at night but rarely meet the night staff, so consider putting up photos with the night staff's names, and ensure that the day staff provide names and contact details of night staff so relatives can call and receive reassurance.

Night-time staff can feel overlooked in terms of support and training, so ensure that they have training needs identified, plus assistance to do their very valuable job to the best of their ability.

Adapted from My Home Life issue 9: Care Home Staff Bulletin: Quality of life at night (www.myhomelifemovement.org/resources/)

A HOME TO LIVE IN NOT EXIST IN

The best care homes I have visited have been those with a family atmosphere, where so often residents will tell me how happy they are and how much the staff mean to them. I am touched by this open, natural response, interaction of staff, residents and relatives, and the establishment of a truly welcoming, adaptable community. I am also aware in these happy homes that much thought has gone into the physical environment and care taken to ensure that the layout of communal areas provides areas of privacy and for people to interact. Seats are arranged not in a stark circle in a lounge where people just stare at each other, but are grouped in smaller, sociable settings. These provide a more natural, less institutionalised environment and greater opportunities for connection. Paintings, lighting, soft furnishings are often tailored around the choices of the residents, allowing again for a sense of positive contribution to the running of the home as a joint community.

THE TEN EDEN ALTERNATIVE PRINCIPLES

I was privileged to be joint keynote speaker with Dr Bill Thomas at a conference in Denmark a few years back. He is an inspirational man who established the Eden Alternative as a way of improving and humanising care homes. I am delighted that they use my films in their trainings. I will use his principles as a recap to this chapter on creating a life worth living for our elders.

1. The three plagues of loneliness, helplessness and boredom account for the bulk of suffering among our elderly.
2. An elder-centred community commits to creating a human habitat where life revolves around close and continuing contact with plants, animals and children. It is these relationships that provide the young and old alike with a pathway to a life worth living.
3. Loving companionship is the antidote to loneliness. Elders deserve easy access to human and animal companionship.
4. An elder-centred community creates opportunity to give as well as receive care. This is the antidote to helplessness.
5. An elder-centred community imbues daily life with variety and spontaneity by creating an environment in which unexpected and unpredictable interactions and happenings can take place. This is the antidote to boredom.
6. Meaningless activity corrodes the human spirit. The opportunity to do things that we find meaningful is essential to human health.

7. Medical treatment should be the servant of genuine human caring, never its master.

8. An elder-centred community honours its elders by de-emphasising top-down bureaucratic authority, seeking instead to place the maximum possible decision-making authority into the hands of the elders or into the hands of those closest to them.

9. Creating an elder-centred community is a never-ending process. Human growth must never be separated from human life.

10. Wise leadership is the lifeblood of any struggle against the three plagues. For it, there is no substitute.

www.edenalternative.co.uk

~

'Without interest you lose everything.'
Solon (630-655 BC)

CHAPTER 5

Heartfelt Communication

Communication is so much more than an exchange of information. It is the means by which we express our thoughts, feelings, hopes and aspirations. It may be a glance, a touch of the hand or a smile that connects us to another human being, banishing loneliness and a sense of isolation.

The interaction with those in your care can be so rewarding. And it's important to examine how we connect, relate and communicate with ourselves and others. Yet I have discovered that communication and connection with those who are elderly or dying is often uncharted territory in training. So I am making a film, *Reach me*, that demonstrates and inspires ways to communicate through words, expression, touch, song, music, rhythm, and through shared silence. This chapter, too, will provide tools to remove the barriers between us, to enable greater opportunities of comfort and connection.

Creating links

HOW ARE YOU?

At the start of my keynote addresses to caring professionals I always ask the audience, 'How are you?' I throw this out to individuals in the audience too; sometimes this startles them and there are giggles of embarrassment. I laugh with them and persevere. Most people then say, 'I am fine', which is a typical English response. I ask them the question again: 'No, how are you *really*, I want to know because I care. *How are you?*' Some will then answer, 'I am tired', 'I am depressed', 'I am anxious'. This honesty in communication is vital if we are to help the mind, body and spirit of an individual. So, as a carer, when you ask someone how they are do you really want to know, do you really care?

If someone asks you how *you* are, do you respond honestly or with a glib, non-committal 'I'm fine'? (I like this humorous interpretation of what 'fine' means: 'Fed up, Irritated, Needy and Emotional'!) If we are unable to answer honestly when someone asks us about our wellbeing, how can we expect others to do the same? We miss the opportunity to create a link of empathy – a moment of humour, perhaps. Look deeper, maintain eye contact and ask, 'How are you? I really want to know, I care.'

If someone is putting out feelers to create a link with you by asking you the same, don't be defensive or dismissive. We English may be private or reserved at times, but please allow yourself to engage with others. Disconnection in care is a dis-ease in itself, allowing for greater feelings of isolation to grow within older people. Share something of yourself, and find more time to talk to people in your care about the things that matter to them – this is an important aspect of any caring role.

WHAT'S IN A NAME?

It's important to find out how the person in your care would prefer to be addressed. Some people may wish to be called by a formal title; others may prefer a more casual approach. Each individual preference should be catered for, because being over-familiar to certain people can be interpreted as disrespectful; being too formal with others may create a barrier. It is about getting the balance right – and doing this by simply asking!

In my workshops I like to discuss with participants the significance of their name: where it comes from, its meaning, whether they have always been known by it, any associations with it, and how they now like to be known. This helps to emphasise the importance of addressing others correctly. When you ask these questions of those you care for, it creates an interesting connection. Consider creating a book of names and their meanings so that staff and those you care for can explore this topic.

EXERCISES TO CONNECT WITH YOUR FEELINGS

Creating stronger links with those in your care often involves examining your own wounds and fears. Understanding and knowing who you are and clearing your own emotional blockages can help you strengthen your connection to others.

I often ask participants in my workshops to nominate the colour that best represents the mood they are in at the moment. It is fascinating to hear how others express themselves visually, and how much is communicated by their sharing of their colours. Consider asking an older person this question, and telling them in turn what colour you are feeling that day and why. Points of contact like this help provide a link, as well as greater understanding of the individual. You can check on the older person throughout the day and see if their colour has changed and why.

You can also use a sound to represent how you are feeling right now. If you do this with a group of people you might hear a choral masterpiece of blending and harmonising, or a chaotic cacophony! Either is good, for you are connecting through sound.

The following exercise gives you permission to relax, so many people in my workshops drink this up like nectar. Consider sharing this exercise with those you care for. It is always good to share time like this together, to share the silence.

Breathe, relax, close your eyes. Go into the stillness. Contemplate emerging thoughts and feelings with emotional stability. Sometimes we run from ourselves, or from others. We are so busy and stressed that we lose the connection with our own life. Breathe, be with yourself for a few moments. Feel how good it is to be connected to yourself, even for a few brief moments. Breathe; enjoy this moment of 'you time'.

When I wake up in the morning, to ensure I am fully returned from my sleep state, and just because it makes me smile, I always say to myself in my head, 'Good morning, Amanda, how are you feeling today?' Some days I might be the only person who asks how I am, so I start the day with an inbuilt caring welcome!

It is very important to check in with yourself during the day, to create a link with yourself, to see how you are doing and make adjustments where necessary. You have to be mindful of your own self-care, to ensure a balance between work, rest and play.

Thoughtful interaction

In my workshops I try to encourage thoughtfulness and consideration in communication. One method is getting carers to role play different scenarios. For example, as a response to someone pressing the call bell, instead of responding by saying something like: 'What do you want now? You just called the bell a few minutes ago – give us a break!' – which of course makes an older person feel vulnerable – I ask the participants to react courteously. Good manners are necessary and valuable in life in general, but particularly in caring situations. Unfortunately, manners can readily fly out the window when a carer is stressed or an older person is in pain. But the importance of respectful behaviour between both parties must not be underestimated.

INCLUDE OTHERS

When carrying out a range of tasks with older people, it helps to include them by discussing what you are doing and the reasons why. Don't just hand medication out without explaining what the medication is and why it is being given. People like to know what is happening, but older people can sometimes forget or may not have the confidence to ask. Informing inspires trust and a sense of security.

BREATHE WITH ME

Communication through breathing can give us clues to how another may be feeling, even if they are unable to communicate verbally. Do not underestimate the power of breath to heal, calm and cleanse the body. I have often been able to connect with a distressed person by firstly copying their breathing patterns audibly. Once I have made that connection, I allow my breath to slow down to a more peaceful pace – and very often this connecting and then slowing enables the other person to match their breathing to my calmer pace. Breathing together, as simple as it may sound, can have an extremely positive effect. Try to experiment with this as part of your communication skills.

WITHOUT WORDS

So much of communication does not even involve words, for it is easy to show emotions and feelings through our facial expressions, posture and gestures. When trying to connect with or understand those who have had a stroke, who are unable to speak or move their body, take the time and give the correct attention to decipher the nuances of expression and sounds. If picture cards are used to help those with communication challenges, to enable them to point to their needs for drink or toilet requirements, to indicate pain levels or the need to be moved, please be aware that these could be on a key chain with smaller laminated picture cards rather than a big cumbersome book that can rob some of their dignity and make them feel like a child.

HOLDING HANDS EXERCISE

In my workshops I use this exercise as a form of non-verbal communication and connection. I arrange everyone into a circle and ask them to hold hands and close their eyes. I choose one person who is designated as the first individual to squeeze the hand of the neighbour on his right. As soon as the neighbour feels that squeeze she passes it on by squeezing the hand of the neighbour on her left, and so on and so on for several rounds. I encourage them to get faster and faster at feeling and then passing the squeeze on. There is always much laughter during this form of non-verbal communication. It is a good exercise to try with elders in any care setting, not only for their reflexes but also for the comfort, touch and sense of inclusion that it can generate.

SENSITIVE COMMUNICATION

Remember that sensitivity and privacy are needed when discussing intimate issues. Limiting distractions and competing demands will help you to give and receive information more effectively. I have often come across staff who mistakenly raise their voices when talking to older people without first ascertaining what their hearing capabilities are. Not all old people are deaf!

I have also seen staff communicate with an older person as if they were stupid or incapable of understanding. Older people are wrongly judged as being slow or not 'with it'. You make this mistake at your peril, for some of the sharpest minds I know are those of octogenarians who could argue you under the table! Again, stereotypical thinking limits dignified and effective communication, and we must be aware that people will need individual modes of interaction suited to their requirements.

ON A FINAL NOTE!

Singing and music are wonderful ways of communicating and connecting with others, particularly those with dementia. This is outlined in the Alzheimer's Society website, www.alzheimers.org.uk, where they advocate Singing for the Brain. The power of sound to heal and harmonise is well documented, and music as medicine and thanatology is becoming more acceptable. Singing together produces a wonderful feeling of camaraderie, whether the songs are carols, lullabies, hymns or music hall songs.

I am often asked to sing in care homes and feel very privileged to do so, particularly when I sing to the very frail and dying as they lie in their beds. From the age of ten I thought about working with the dying. I had an overwhelming urge to cure loneliness – I could not bear the thought of someone dying alone. And I still can't. My answer would be to sing at the Royal Hospital and Home for Incurables (as it was then called) and at local care homes and hospices. My school friends thought I was most strange.

Singing has always been part of my life and I have sung the lead in many musicals as an actress, but I have never felt more privileged to sing than during the passing of my grandmother and mother and father, singing back to them the lullabies they sang to me as a child. I have recorded the songs I sang as simple but powerful tracks to calm and soothe those who are facing times of crisis and transition, that they may feel they are not alone. The CD is called *I am near you* and is a combination of song and spoken word. So many elderly people are dying alone, and I hope this CD can be used to provide a missing link when the physical presence of a loved one or carer is not possible. They can listen to the simple human voice as if someone were there in the room, holding their hand and allaying distress.

'Whatever words we utter should be chosen with care for people will hear them and be influenced by them for good or ill.'

Buddha

CHAPTER 6

Compassion in Action

'We believe we are hurt when we don't receive love, but that is not what hurts us. Our pain comes when we do not give love. Mankind was born to love, and our wellbeing depends on our giving love. It is not about what comes back, it's about what goes out.'

Alan Cohen

'Love in care is not a dirty word.'

Amanda Waring

What are the differences between empathy, compassion and love? Empathy is like a map that tells us where we can go and what we can do in different areas; empathy tells us how another feels so we can better judge what we say or do without hurting those we look after. Empathy is a starting point, a skill you can build upon that can lead to the emergence of compassion and love. Observation and listening intently become critical skills, as does maintaining a non-judgemental perspective.

I see compassion and love being facets of wisdom. So when

we act from wisdom, compassion and love, our actions will be effective; we will not act inappropriately, we will act in a way which benefits everyone and promotes understanding and healing. Compassion can simply mean kindness. It can mean patience, generosity, respect, sympathy and understanding. It is unconditional love.

These qualities of compassion and empathy can transform ourselves as well as others, providing us with a vocational aspect to caring as we become unafraid to connect with our heart.

The Janki Foundation for Global Health Care promotes the following beliefs:

'We acknowledge a patient's illness, we sense how they feel, we try to understand how it affects them, yet with compassion we do not become emotionally involved. We are engaged, yet detached. We are standing back and looking on with kindness. By showing compassion in this way in the healthcare setting, it allows us to be compassionate without suffering from "compassion fatigue" or "burnout". We can do this by developing the skill of compassionate listening.'

We also need to understand the importance of having compassion for ourselves.

In my training sessions I use the following quote by Sogyal Rinpoche, the author of *The Tibetan Book of Living and Dying*:

'The moment you feel compassion welling up inside you, don't brush it aside, don't shrug it off and try quickly to return to "normal", don't be afraid of the feeling or be embarrassed by it, allow yourself to be distracted from it, or let it run aground in apathy. But be vulnerable, use that quick, bright uprush of compassion; focus on it, go deep into your heart and meditate on it, develop it, enhance and deepen it.'

WINDOWS OF THE SOUL EXERCISE

In my workshops I like to explore that feeling of compassion expressed in Rinpoche's quote. I pair up carers to sit opposite each other and look into each other's eyes. There are always giggles to begin with, but these settle in time as I speak the words below while the carers maintain eye contact:

Look into the eyes of your partner. Allow that feeling of compassion to shine through your eyes. You are not having to fix anything, say anything or do anything, but just maintain a soft gaze with your partner. If you feel embarrassed, let that feeling pass, just breathe and *be* with the other person, holding eye contact. How are you feeling? Do you feel a deeper connection with the person opposite you? Can you feel their emotions, their needs? The next time you are listening to an elder in your care, consider this moment of being actively relaxed but fully present. You don't need to provide solutions or answers; just allowing yourself to fully be with that person is enough.

The response to this exercise has been quite profound. Carers discovered more empathy and compassion for themselves and for others. We so rarely look into the eyes of another, to see who they are and to see ourselves reflected back.

MEDITATION ON COMPASSION

Sit comfortably and relax. Feel your feet on the ground, your connection to the earth. Allow the muscles of your shoulders and neck to relax ... dissolve the tension into the ground. Let the muscles of your arms and legs feel relaxed ... now your face.

Now focus your attention on your breathing. Let it find its own calm rhythm. Gently breathe in peacefulness and calm, and breathe out any negative feelings.

Allow your mind to slow down. Try to watch your thoughts. Do not judge them as good or bad; they are just thoughts. Acknowledge them and let them go ... they are like clouds in the sky that you can watch drifting past. Beyond the clouds is the deep blueness of the sky. Feel that deep calm of the blue sky ...

Now focus on your own inner calm ... that place deep within yourself that is peaceful, where your inner compassion lies. Here you are patient, tolerant, generous, understanding ... all these qualities are here. They make up your own inner compassion. Experience the feeling of compassion; feel it within you and see it focused as a point ... a point of light ...

Now raise your awareness beyond yourself to a place of infinite peace ... see it first as a small point of light. As you move towards it, it becomes brighter ... it is like an ocean of peace ... a space of calm, of love, of compassion. You feel connected; part of that ocean of deep peace and love. It surrounds you like a cloak, it fills you up, absorbing every part of you with a comfortable warmth.

Rest in that feeling of being loved. It is like energy ... a vibration ... a light filling you until you overflow ...

Now slowly move away from the ocean as a point of light. You still have the memory of being loved, and can reconnect any time you wish ...

Gradually become aware of your body. Feel your feet on the ground ...

Adapted from the meditation on the Janki Foundation website www.jankifoundation.org

EMPATHY AND COMPASSION EXERCISE

Moving towards a more compassionate model of care requires all health and social care practitioners to take as full account as possible of an older person's individuality in responding to the range of psychological, spiritual, social and physical needs that affects their quality of life. For older people, and particularly those with dementia, it is important to have those who can walk alongside them and accept them for who they are at that moment.

To inspire compassion, empathy, and understanding of the consequences of physical disability, boredom and loneliness, I read out the following in my workshops, asking participants to close their eyes as I do so.

Imagine that you have experienced some trauma that has left you unable to move any part of your body except your head. You are now living in a nursing home, and you are dependent on others for your most basic needs. The carers have given you your breakfast, cleaned you up, dressed you and put you in a wheelchair. They have wheeled you in front of the nurses' station. All you can see is the top of a nurse's head as she leans down to write. Occasionally you can see people scurrying by as they go about their duties; what you see is mostly feet and knees. You can hear the phone ringing and the nurse answering it, staff chattering and laughing, the intercom blaring and the floor polisher roaring. Now imagine that you have been sitting here for an hour ... now two hours ... You are so tired, you are no longer able to hold up your head ...

Imagine if this was your life for two months ... two years ...

(Adapted from the Eden Alternative)

By doing this short exercise, most participants feel motivated to engage more with those in their care and be mindful of how long they leave others alone and ignored. Meaningless time-passing corrodes the spirit, so both planned and spontaneous activities – always compatible with individual preferences, lifestyle, interests and capabilities – need to be instigated to prevent boredom, loss of hope, helplessness and loneliness. Having a focus only on medical needs ignores the spiritual richness of elderhood. Short sharp shock tactics, as I use with my films, can be powerful aids to refocus you on what is important: the experience and quality of life of those you care for.

THE CARERS BEATITUDE

I use this to remind carers of how the practice of compassion can be so valued by those you care for; the effects are tangible and appreciated.

> Blessed are they who understand
> My faltering steps and shaking hand.
>
> Blessed they who know my ears today
> Must strain to catch the things they say.
>
> Blessed are they with a cheery smile
> Who stop for a chat for a little while.
>
> Blessed are they who never say
> 'You've told me that story twice today.'
>
> Blessed are they who make it known
> That I am loved, respected and not alone.

Adapted from 'Beatitudes for Friends
of the Aged' *by Esther Mary Walker*

'If you want others to be happy, practice compassion. If you want to be happy, practice compassion.'

Dalai Lama XIV, *The Art of Happiness: A Handbook for Living*

CHAPTER 7

Dementia Care

Which would you prefer, to exist or to live?

Living must not be about mere existence, but about actively thriving and flourishing within the capabilities of the individual. For those working with people who have dementia, a more creative and feelings-based approach is needed to understand the 'lived world' of the person with dementia. If staff are not trained in specialist enabling and communication skills, it is likely that the individual with dementia will be misunderstood and that their emotional, occupational and social needs will not be met.

Colour, spontaneity, variety, and catching opportunities for magic moments through engagement, human connection and social interaction can make all the difference to those with dementia. We need you as care givers to be inspired to gently enter into the world of people locked away or withdrawn into their own reality.

Understanding senile dementia

To provide the best quality care that we can for those with dementia we must understand that dementia is not an unchangeable illness where nothing further can be done, it is a *disability* which is made up of someone's unique life history, general health, personality, specific damage to a part of the brain and the attitudes of those caring for them. Realising that dementia is a disability lets us know that, through treatment and support, well-being can be supported or even improved, and that the duty of good care is about preserving the person behind the disability.

When caring for those with dementia it is vital that we have an understanding of the psychological as well as the physical aspects of this disease. This chapter explores the interior world of those with dementia, to enable us to realise that all behaviour is meaningful and needs to be understood, not just managed, and that emotional needs are as important as physical needs.

'SLIPPING AWAY A BIT AT A TIME'

The author Terry Pratchett, who has a type of early-onset Alzheimer's, wrote in an article for the *Daily Mail*: 'I am slipping away a bit at a time, and all I can do is watch it happen.'

In her book *Insight into Dementia* (CWR Publishing, 2010), Rosemary Hurtley writes: 'Senile dementia of the Alzheimer's type is a progressive global impairment of intellectual, then daily, living skills, slowly eroding abilities over a period of years, arising from changes in the brain, plaques of protein in brain tissue and tangles of abnormal nerve fibres in cells. This is the most common type of dementia.'

The dementia journey can be a long and hard one for the sufferer and the carer alike. Once a diagnosis of dementia has been given, people are sadly likely to experience a profound sense of loss:

- A loss of intellectual capacity – short term memory loss, making logical connections
- Reduced communication ability due to poor concentration and language difficulties
- A loss of independence – problems with getting lost, requiring supervision in activities

These losses combine to create the conditions for frustration, depression, poor self-esteem, fear of failure, and anxiety about what the future might hold. Self-esteem is vital for maintaining relationships and one's sense of place in the world. It is important for someone with dementia to receive reassurances and to stay connected with familiar activities that help create a sense of identity, belonging and connection. Helping them feel valued, to feel that their life is important and that they can still contribute, are vital ways to prevent the deep sense of aloneness that can overwhelm someone challenged with dementia.

I have made a short film of the following poem by my friend the highly esteemed nurse Pat Duff OBE. It perfectly illustrates the sense of loss, and is used in my trainings to deepen the understanding of the world of someone with dementia. Understanding helps us not to judge but to validate feelings, empathise and then assist where we can. How can we reach people from their world rather than ours? What could we do to alleviate their pain and anxiety?

> It comes again relentlessly
> The shredding of my thoughts
> The disappearing sense of me
> And who I am or was

The window opens inches wide
Behind the blanks of dark
I fear the breaking cordless sash
That shuts me out at once

My anxious capsule gripping tight
So seldom yields away
My lucid moments filled with fear
A constant crippling pain

The gentle aura of your touch
The respite of your hands
My present moments feel the calm
And I know who I am.

Pat Duff OBE

As I like to use a multi-media approach to helping others engage deeply with the experience of those they care for, in 2011 I made an experimental CD recording, 'I am calling you'. Here I sing the anguish and searing pain of someone with dementia as they go through a very dark emotional space, where they seem unreachable, to demonstrate the locked-in pain that can occur when confusion reigns. As the track progresses the carer's voice and presence slowly helps return them 'home'. And though this track makes uncomfortable listening, it powerfully portrays the interior world of those challenged with dementia.

IF *YOU* HAD DEMENTIA

Try to walk in the shoes of a person with dementia to fully understand the challenges and stresses they face. This will help you grasp their specific needs and the positive steps you can take to support them.

- If *you* had dementia you would probably have problems with ideas, words, speech and possibly hearing, as well as repeating yourself. You would suffer from confusion of people, time or place, have difficulties in instigating and continuing a conversation, and trouble with making decisions, often forgetting mid-flow what is being talked about. You would find yourself dwelling in the past and over-reacting. The carers who look after you need patience and reassurance to be able to meet you in your present, along your own spectrum of 'time travel'.

- If *you* had dementia you would experience mood swings, so those who care for you need to be aware of the nuances of your behaviour and to identify if you are being influenced by physical pain or emotional pain, or both.

- If *you* had dementia you would experience increasing problems understanding what is being said to you and what is going on around you. You may find it very difficult to communicate with others and may gradually lose your speech or cry out from time to time. Those caring for you need to remember that verbal language is only one way of communicating; they need to take the time to observe your expressions and body language, which will provide them with clues as to how you are feeling.

- If *you* had dementia you would possibly also have a visual or hearing impairment, and so be frustrated at experiencing further barriers. You would feel an isolation due to a lack of awareness of your environment, which could lead to you having a fear of falling or of having accidents. You would have an all-pervading sense of anxiety. You would need carers to reach you, support and reassure you as you feel yourself suffering from withdrawal, having less opportunity for participation, and reduced involvement in activities. You would need carers to give emotional and practical support to retain your interests within your capabilities, to include you in positive social encounters, and to provide sufficient activity choices and meaningful roles.

- If *you* had dementia, could you see why your behaviour may be unco-operative, and wouldn't you rather your carers understood the underlying reasons rather than force medication on you?

(Adapted from Insight into Dementia *by Rosemary Hurtley)*

Given what you have just experienced walking in another's shoes, will your perceptions and tolerance levels change?

EFFECTS OF DEMENTIA ON FAMILIES

The diagnosis of dementia can be devastating for relatives, and the effects can be cataclysmic. They can involve anger, anxiety, frustration, loneliness, tiredness, guilt and grief. Family members also have to deal with the potential stigma attached to dementia and how different people react to the diagnosis. This was a friend of mine's experience: 'When my dad was diagnosed with dementia, people who had known him for many years would ask about him, but when I said "Why don't you pop over and visit?" it was so obvious they were uncomfortable with the idea. I felt like screaming, "He's the same bloody person you know, he could do with the company. He just can't do some things any more; but so what, he still loves a joke and a drink. Don't shut him out because you feel uncomfortable – it's not catching, you know. Don't stop being his friend."'

Relatives need gentle support and understanding; if they are supported they can better help you support their loved ones with dementia.

HOW TIMES HAVE CHANGED

It is good to see the changing attitudes towards dementia care within care settings. The table below is encouraging to see how times are changing and acts as a stark reminder to not slip back into former outdated modes of care. Examine your place of care and see if you may be inadvertently practising the old culture of care and be inspired to shift this into the new culture of dementia care.

Old culture of dementia care	New culture of dementia care
Dementia is an undemanding field to work in; few skills are needed	Dementia is an exciting area of practice requiring high levels of skill
Dementia is a progressive and degenerative disease and no action can be taken to make a difference	Dementia is a disability and wellbeing depends on the quality of care provided
The expertise lies only with doctors and scientists	Care-givers are experts
Research is based on cures and treatments	Research should aim to develop quality care
Care culture of 'them and us'	Staff seen as equals
Care is limited to meeting physical needs and emphasising what a person could not do/would decline	Care priority is to address emotional and physical needs; intervention is based on what a person can do
Problem behaviour needs to be managed/controlled	All behaviour has meaning, which needs to be understood before responses are based on underlying needs and feelings
Caregivers should put aside personal feelings and concentrate on the job at hand	Caregivers need to be in touch with their own feelings and management needs to enable development

(*The above is a summary based on* New Culture of Dementia Care, *edited by Tom Kitwood and Sue Benson, Hawker Publications, 1995*)

Communicating with people with dementia

COMMUNICATION CHALLENGES

Some specific difficulties encountered when attempting to communicate with people with dementia can include:

- They confuse the past with the present reality
- They have problems remembering normal routines, services used, appointments
- They have problems communicating thoughts and feelings
- They have varying awareness levels
- There is physical and social environment disorientation
- They have reduced insight and awareness of problems
- They have difficulties with memory recall
- They repeat themselves
- Their conversation slows down
- They are unable to convey much information
- They say things that are not based on the reality of the listener
- They have difficulties with reading or writing
- There is poor eye contact

(Adapted from the Alzheimer's Society, 2009)

RUNNING COMMENTARY

Using a running commentary when communicating with someone with dementia can improve their ability to navigate and orientate themselves. Remind them of what has just happened, tell them what is happening now and what is about to happen. Use simple but clear language. It is also important to ensure that eye contact is made before any personal care activities.

RISING TO THE CHALLENGES

Any one of the following problems could become an issue when you are communicating with someone with dementia. So let's identify some actions to take.

Repetitive behaviour: repetitive speech is common, as the person forgets from one minute to the next.

Action: make sure there is a time gap between questions and reassure the person, rephrasing their words back to them. Ensure needs have been met. Provide distraction: offer something else to see, hear or do.

Losing things/making accusations of theft: this can occur in the early stages of dementia.

Action: carers should not get into a confrontation, and should remember that this can be related to, or a mirror of, deeper losses or previous experiences. Carers can ask them where they last saw the object, or ascertain if they have a favourite hiding place. It is a good idea to keep replacements (of keys, etc) and to check wastepaper baskets and bins before emptying them.

Hallucinations: the person may misinterpret what they see or hear, such as hearing people talking in the room or seeing a figure at the end of the bed.

Action: try not to confront or contradict what they have seen or heard. Use a calm and comforting voice to reassure them and distract their attention to something real. Some medication may be the cause so seek appropriate medical advice, but be aware that something as simple as deteriorating hearing and eyesight can contribute to any confusion so ensure checkups and assessments are done.

Aggressive outbursts
Action: find out where possible what has triggered the outburst, which can often be due to loss of control and frustration with communication problems. Divert them to a calming activity and remember not to take aggression personally. But if violence occurs, seek professional help to manage this behaviour.

Loss of motivation: this can be due to a loss of confidence, interest and ability to initiate an activity.
Action: Give verbal prompts such as 'Can you help me with . . . ?' or 'I'd love your assistance with . . .' alongside physical prompts such as pointing or miming or handing the person the tool for the job.

Difficulty keeping up with familiar routines
Action: gently take over related responsibilities as abilities diminish, but involve the person wherever possible, encouraging them to undertake familiar, simple activities.

Poor communication
Action: stop, observe, listen, engage. Try to observe the person's mood, breathing and movement; listen to words and metaphors that may give clues to what they are trying to express. Use your imagination to enter their world and then engage with their emotions and needs. Communicate using verbal and non-verbal methods. We need to be aware too of the importance of the use of touch and the tone of our voice.

Difficulty getting dressed
Action: occupational therapists are so helpful for advice on daily living support, but remember not to overwhelm someone with dementia with too much clutter or choice, which can confuse them further. Consider using Velcro to replace buttons, and lay

the clothes out in the order they are to be put on. Use of labels, pictures and whole outfits together provides simple choices.

Falling
Action: remove loose mats, encourage the person to pick their feet up and take longer strides, but do not push or pull the individual. Patterned carpets can cause confusion, as can the depth of stairs, so consider marking edges with bright masking tape. Ensure there is a dimmer switch or night light to assist orientation and reduce anxiety.

MEDICATION VERSUS COUNSELLING

'Medical treatment should be the servant of genuine human caring, never its master.'
Dr Bill Thomas, founder of the Eden Alternative

When I talk at conferences I make a plea to stop overmedicating the elderly. Medication, particularly of those with dementia, may be given for behaviour which is challenging to others, such as aggression, shouting, delusions and psychotic symptoms. But this behaviour can be down to communication difficulties and a misinterpretation of needs. Latest evidence suggests that powerful sedative drugs are used too early, without first examining underlying emotional needs that require careful and dedicated unravelling to heal or release the source of the agitation.

Validation therapy and deeper forms of counselling can help address loss, bereavement and traumatic events that can easily rise to the surface out of context as a person with dementia moves between different worlds and time frames. Powerful tranquilising drugs that have been used to treat symptoms rather than the cause of behaviour have serious negative side effects such as reducing mobility, increasing the likelihood of a stroke and doubling cognitive decline. Obviously this drug-orientated approach 'zombifies' older people and is not an acceptable therapy in so many instances. It should be used only in severe cases as a last resort.

Promoting wellbeing in dementia

> 'Among those whom I like or admire, I can find no common denominator; but among those whom I love, I can: all of them make me laugh.'
>
> **W.H. Auden**

ALLOW THE UNEXPECTED

Activating wellness in dementia requires carers to be playful and emotionally in tune. Carers should be encouraged to work with the senses in a therapeutic way. A sense of fun and spontaneity, and joining in the moment, are gifts that can change the atmosphere and lift the spirits. A range of objects displayed at different levels creates a natural environment where spontaneity can occur. This might include themed sets of material items and memorabilia – consider the interests and themes that are most evident in the lives of those you care for – which can be changed around often to promote different thoughts, language and memories. They can be laid out on tables, shelves, along corridors, bringing the richness and variety of the world into their personal space.

CULTIVATE EMPATHY

Rather than just having an understanding of what people with dementia might need, it is also important to ensure that they have those who can walk alongside them as they try to express themselves, accepting them for who they are at that moment. We need to learn to be present in their reality by stepping into their shoes, armed with as much knowledge as possible about the person, their background and the things that matter most to them. It is easy to make wrong judgements or even try to 'fix' the confusion rather than relieve their tensions and fears. People with dementia can be very poetic and see the world in a more metaphorical and symbolic way as they move through different time zones and worlds, which can be daunting to a carer. But it can also be liberating, inspiring, challenging and even exciting at times. Be open to the experience of learning from your fellow time travellers; it may be a bumpy but exhilarating and insightful ride. Our lives and perspectives can be enriched through caring for those with dementia.

MEMORIES AS MEDICINE

The person with dementia sees the world differently, similar to the faculties of a child but with the memories of an entire life. Focusing on distant memories can sometimes be a means of escape from pain or anguish, becoming a coping mechanism to tune out the current reality.

To experience this for yourself, focus on a tense part of your body and close your eyes; feel the discomfort and really focus on this for a few moments. Now think of a happy memory and remember the joy, the excitement. After a minute refocus on the previous discomfort – has anything changed, are you less tense than you were?

Encourage relatives to bring in photographs showing important people, places, events or interests with explanatory notes or captions. Life histories provide an opportunity to see individuals as multi-faceted people and provide valuable information for planning activities. Memory boxes are a useful tool as well. For example, you could make a memory box for someone who liked gardening and the outdoor life by including objects such as seed packets, old gardening gloves, fir cones, flower pictures, herbs and floral fragrant sachets, recordings of birds singing, music associated with flowers and gardens. Get creative! These boxes can be developed for group interests as well as one to one sessions.

I recommend reading *Contented Dementia* by Oliver James (Vermilion, 2009). It's a very useful explanation of the SPECAL (Specialised Early Care for Alzheimer's) method which promotes a way of using the past to make sense of the present.

RULES OF ENGAGEMENT

Assessing what individuals are interested in and what they are able to do is essential for person-centred quality of life plans. Use the questions below to help you consider how you might assist those in you care to engage in something they might enjoy doing.

- *Personality*: what type of person are they?
- *Biography*: what kind of life roles have they enjoyed? How can they be encouraged to maintain a role in ways that are important to them in their current community? What have they enjoyed in the past? What might they like to do to provide continuity with the past and engagement in the present?
- *Cognitive abilities*: what levels of assistance are required to help them to follow through an activity? Do they have the attention span to sustain interest/concentration?
- *Social factors*: do they like company, and if so how much? Do they prefer to spend time alone? What type of

company do they prefer (kindred spirits, shared interests and background, etc)? Can they cope with social situations, for example taking turns, contributing to a group?

- *Physical factors*: what are their movement skills, coordination, strength, physical condition, levels of pain? How is their sense of balance; do they suffer frequent falls? What are their sensory abilities?

Personal care for people with dementia

BATHING PEOPLE WITH DEMENTIA

Bathing can be a source of stress if it is carried out in a task-orientated way. People may not associate bathing with washing and may not understand or recognise the sensation of water. It can be seen as an invasion of privacy and dignity if not attended to sensitively. If arthritic or other pain is unattended it can cause anxiety. Here are some tips to make bathing a more enjoyable experience:

- Bath time can be enjoyable and relaxing and should not be rushed.
- Find out from the older person or their advocate or family if they have any preferences, habits or anxieties around bath time. Taking into consideration a person's lifelong habits will individualise the bathing experience and help to prevent stress or anxiety.
- The environment should be relaxing and homely, incorporating principles of good design. Soft relaxing music or aromatherapy can help some people. Check that the temperature is comfortable. Let the older person hear the sound of running water

- Use good communication: identify yourself, ask permission, and explain instructions carefully, using short sentences and emphasising key words, accompanied by demonstration if necessary. Use body language and gesture with appropriate tone of voice to support what you are saying.
- Provide the level of support appropriate to their capabilities; for instance, recognising objects and what they are used for can be a problem for some people. Start an activity such as using a flannel, demonstrating the washing movement to prompt memory. To determine cognitive level and amount of support needed, use a simple cognitive assessment such as the Pool Activity Level (PAL) instrument (see *Reducing Stress-related Behaviours in People with Dementia* by Chris Bonner, Jessica Kingsley Publishers, London 2005).
- This intimate time provides an opportunity to gently move and exercise stiff and painful joints in warm water.
- Always explain what is going to happen next, using simple, respectful language. Use reminiscence and small talk to make the person feel included and involved.
- Don't forget to consider feelings of modesty.
- Document what works well in the care plan.

EATING DIFFICULTIES

An older person with dementia will have additional difficulties such as being able to express wishes, recognise food or eating utensils and remember how to use them. They may have swallowing difficulties. Some people are easily distracted and restless and have difficulty sitting down for more than a few minutes. Altered senses of smell, taste and vision may also affect appetite. In addition, some medication, discomfort or pain can affect the desire to eat.

Below are some suggestions that may help people with dementia at mealtimes:

- Assess level of independence, preferences for food and the physical and social environment.
- Involve the family if necessary to find out about eating habits and preferences.
- Encouraging social interaction at mealtimes can improve the enjoyment of the meal. Make sure the social mix around the table is compatible. A level of formality at table might encourage a person to eat as a social activity.
- When helping someone to eat, give them your full attention, facing them and talking to them and including simple explanations in full view. Allow enough time to chew and swallow food. Encourage continuity with carers who know the older person well and are sensitive to their habits (key worker).
- Avoid unnecessary noise and background distractions, although the use of music and nature sounds can encourage eating.
- Loss of senses and changes related to ageing can be supplemented with use of spices and additional flavour and appetising smells.
- Use of regular finger foods and snacks can help when main meals require supplementing to satisfy energy needs, particularly if a person is constantly on the move.
- Stimulate memory by providing familiar food, linked to childhood memories.
- Serve one course at a time, using small portions on a plate. Too much food on a plate can affect appetite.
- Ensure that there are clear contrasts between plates, cups and table to help those who find it difficult to distinguish between foreground and background. Avoid heavily patterned cloths.

- Only give assistance when needed, encouraging older people to do as much for themselves as possible.
- If there are swallowing difficulties, gently stroke the larynx in an upward motion to encourage a swallowing reflex. Refer to a speech and language therapist for advice on thickeners and complex swallowing problems.

(Adapted from Reducing Stress-related Behaviours in People with Dementia *by Chris Bonner.)*

Exploring activities for people with dementia

Stage of dementia	Potential activities
Early dementia	Board games, physically competitive games/sports, quizzes, discussions, end-product tasks, structured crafts, work-type activity. Use memory and orientation aids, crib cards, timetable.
Early to middle dementia	Music, dance, drama, art, poetry, reminiscence, story telling, festive/seasonal and spiritual activities.
Middle to late dementia	Movement, massage, cooking, stacking, rummaging, dolls and soft toys, balls, exercise, bubbles, balloons, gardening, folding , polishing, wiping, sweeping, 'clowning'. Involve all the senses.
Late dementia	Singing, rocking, holding, non-verbal communication, smiling, stroking. Reflex responses to direct stimulation.

PRINCIPLES FOR PROVIDING ACTIVITIES

- Activities help to provide a structure to the day and give a sense of belonging.

- Activities provide opportunities to reduce restlessness and agitation plus opportunities for both verbal and non-verbal communication.
- Activities should be directed at reducing ill-being and raising wellbeing.
- A person's ability to engage in an activity will change over the course of dementia, so it is important to regularly review which activities the person responds to.
- Aim to support the feelings behind what the person is saying, rather than disputing what they actually are saying (for instance, if they are talking about something that happened to them many years ago).

PRACTICAL GUIDE TO SUCCESSFUL USE OF ACTIVITIES

- Find out what stage and level of function the resident is at by using the PAL Checklist (Pool Activity Level instrument – see note on page 90).
- Find out as much as you can about the resident's past, their life story, interests, preferences, and personality type.
- Encouraging the person or group to be spontaneous and express themselves will promote liveliness and enjoyment.
- Give as many opportunities for communicating, interacting and relating to others as possible.
- Use more sensory and non-verbal ways of communicating in the later stages of dementia.
- Be flexible in your choice of activity, and choose activities that you and the resident enjoy.
- Try to use your imagination and intuition, adopting a natural and playful approach.
- Focus on abilities rather than problems, using either group or one to one approaches, remembering that if the person is very impaired an individual approach will be needed.

- Successful approaches include a lively, joyous and humorous manner using lots of non-verbal communication and stimulating sight. Use movement and repetition within tasks, which should be short and familiar to the resident.
- Provide a consistent routine, maintain rituals and minimise distractions.
- To provide reassurance, use the resident's name frequently, remind them what has just taken place, remind them what is about to happen.
- A match must be made between the individual abilities and the demands of the task, that is, a balance between challenge and skill. If the task is too challenging the resident may become anxious, but if it is insufficiently challenging they may become bored.

IDEAS FOR PEOPLE WITH MODERATE DEMENTIA TO ENJOY

Here are some creative ideas for activities that anyone can do; most are failure free and therefore useful for people with moderate dementia to enjoy.

Vegetable printing: Various objects can be dipped in PVA or poster paints. Sliced vegetables, either natural or with cut patterns, or polystyrene, sponge, cork or other objects can be used for printing. Use fabric paints for fabric printing.

Doodling: Give the pupil a felt pen and paper and encourage free movement over the paper in a continuous line, preferably with eyes closed. Always encourage a sense of enjoyment.

Splodging: Blobs of watercolour paint or coloured inks can be dropped onto a damp piece of paper. Shapes can be drawn later with a brush, if the pupil is able, to add meaning to the splodges.

Water painting: Use a wide brush, mixed non-toxic quality watercolours in bright colours, short small sealable jars (taller jars are difficult for people with limited arm movements to retrieve brushes from) and a piece of paper (a roll of quality lining paper will last a long time) which has been wetted. Put the paper on gloss-painted hardboard sheets, about two feet square, and use sponges to wipe away any excess water. Bring in greenery and seasonal flowers to place on the table.

Finger painting: Put primary colours onto the fingers of each hand and 'play the piano' to the sound of music – gently flowing, with an occasional lively part.

Marbling: Half fill a shallow plastic tray or trough with water (old roasting tins or plastic cat trays are ideal). Open bottles of waterproof ink. Use a dipper to drop the ink gently onto the surface of water, or touch the water with an ink-filled brush. Lay the paper on the top of the water for a few seconds to absorb the colour and remove. Lay out to dry. The end product can be used for a range of different projects such as decorating rims of paper plates before a picture is placed in the centre, plastic cups (using a mixture of oil paints with white spirit on water), flowerpots (first preparing with white emulsion paint to seal).

Straw blowing: Non-waterproof ink or watercolour paints can be blobbed on paper. Blow on the blobs through straws.

Stencil painting: Doilies and other shapes can be used as stencils with paint or felt pens.

Rubbing: This can be done over bark or objects stuck down on card. Use a wax crayon to rub over the paper to make a print.

Rubber stamping: Use rubber shapes or images stuck onto a wood block and a stamp pad.

Combing: Use a mixture of colour paint, a Polycell double strength mixture and water. Use a comb shape cut out of stiff card of desired shape. Draw patterns with the comb onto paper which has been prepared by brushing on the paint and Polycell mixture.

Templates: Make templates for people to draw round, or do this yourself, depending on ability levels.

IDEAS FOR ACTIVITIES FOR LATER STAGES OF DEMENTIA

Encourage spontaneity as much as you can.

Provide:
- Rummaging-boxes with a range of interesting objects, fabrics, items of interest, objects or things of particular personal significance.
- Treasure chests containing some interesting, surprising things.
- Dressing up items such as hats, gloves, scarves.
- Coloured paper and wool for tearing, winding, folding, making collages.
- Poems, large print songs for reading aloud.
- Old items for reminiscence – old clothes, tools, day-to-day memorabilia.

Try to encourage activities such as:
- Helping with domestic activities – laying and wiping tables, dusting, washing up, sorting socks, folding laundry, tidying drawers.
- Work-type activities – folding paper, stuffing envelopes.
- Simple gardening – planting, tending, arranging.
- Natural movement – swaying, using scarves to interpret different types of music.

Other activities:
- Massage – hand and neck, using aromatherapy oils.
- Get families to bring in babies and pets.
- Making and giving gifts.

Remember the important principle is to join people where they are in time and place and consider the world from their perspective.

MUSIC

Music is a powerful and versatile medium which can be used in a variety of interesting and creative ways. It transcends language and taps into memories that often remain longer than verbal ability. It can be calming, motivating, stimulating, relaxing, and can promote singing, self-expression through spontaneous movement and exercise. It can be incorporated into other activities such as reminiscence, quizzes, opening and closing sessions (see page 99), relaxation and discussions. It can be part of a planned or spontaneous activity, passive or active entertainment.

We can communicate through the power of music. Music enriches the brain and nourishes the spirit. Try painting to music. Group members spend time listening to music and using wetted cartridge paper, brushes and watercolours to sweep across the page from left to right, reflecting the music, or to draw a picture reflecting music.

Listening and responding to music is a great stress reliever. People with dementia will show a greater freedom and spontaneity and may wish to get up and move to the music. Think about the age group of the people you care for and discuss the range of music that they enjoyed in their youth. It is also good to introduce new things to people, as not everyone wants to remain in the past. Try to incorporate a variety of music in your sessions, taking into account the range of tastes among residents.

It is easy to make wrong assumptions about what people like or dislike based on stereotypes rather than individual differences. Always observe, trying to be sensitive and respectful to responses, never assuming what people might like.

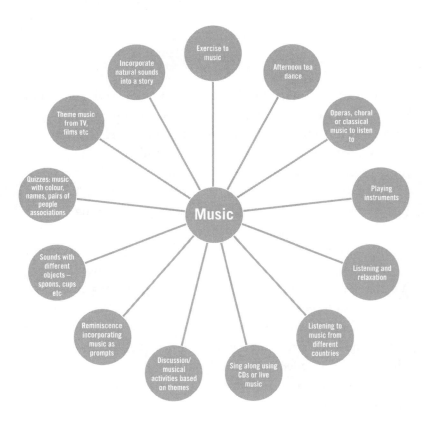

DANCE AND DRAMA

Dance offers a different way of self-expression and creativity which is emotional and aesthetic, providing a personal or a shared experience. Dance uses music working around individuals, reflecting their gestures as dialogue.

A wide range of music and rhythms can be used. A tea dance provides opportunities for expression through music, fun, enjoyment, interaction, movement, reminiscence and body awareness. It taps into movement- and music-memories.

Drama uses an intuitive approach, requiring a full range of communication skills to facilitate activity. Creativity is stimulated along with the senses, providing opportunities for movement expression. It can provide a sense of fun and enjoyment and raise levels of wellbeing. Drama can improve communication and interaction, it stimulates imagination and memory. It does not need to involve learning lines or costumes.

Try to use every avenue of communication, working intuitively, emphasising the use of voice, touch and listening skills. Introduce objects where possible to represent reality, and promote interaction and contact. The benefits include increased motivation, concentration, sensory stimulation and relaxation.

TECHNIQUES FOR USE IN MUSIC, DANCE AND DRAMA

Opening and closing rituals: These can include a theme tune; repetitive movements such as clapping, swaying, rocking, stamping feet, waving scarves to music or rubbing hands; throwing a large soft ball; passing props around for people to pick out from a bag. At the end of a session the ritual could include holding hands and looking around the group saying 'thank you' as an expression of togetherness. Passing round a doll or a teddy bear can make talking via the object easier, and can give permission for cuddling and comforting.

Mime: Body exercises can be used as a warm-up, for example stroking or rubbing hands and different parts of the body, clenching and stretching fingers open. Mime everyday activities such as picking flowers, putting them into a vase, being presented with some flowers, opening a present, brushing teeth. Miming can be done together or individually, with others guessing what the mime is if they are able.

Storymaking: Familiar and favourite stories can be effectively used, or make up a story involving simple movement such as waving, smiling, walking. A large picture can be used to identify why, what, where and when, stimulating use of language; it can also be used to make up a story. Include props, mime and taking roles where possible.

Hats: Using simple props is an effective way of getting attention. Hats can be used with gloves, scarves and costume jewellery (with mirrors available for added enjoyment). Simple mimes can be acted out. Some of these activities can stimulate memories and language skills.

'I have seen deeply demented patients weep or shiver as they listen to music they have never heard before, and I think they can experience the entire range of feelings the rest of us can, and that dementia, at least at these times, is no bar to emotional depth. Once one has seen such responses, one knows that there is still a self to be called upon, even if music, and only music, can do the calling.'

Oliver Sacks, *Musicophilia: Tales of Music and the Brain*

CHAPTER 8

When the Going Gets Tough

Do not underestimate the emotional and physical toll that caring for others can have on us. Caring for another human being offers up many challenges, both emotional and physical, and burnout and stress are so common that it is vital to be aware of your own needs, and to nurture your own mind, body and spirit. Our duty of self-care is of primary importance, but how often do we put ourselves first?

Over the next few pages I will provide you with tools and innovative ideas to relax and restore energy when the going gets tough, and to inspire you to keep on keeping on.

Engage/disengage

Although throughout this book I encourage you to engage with those in your care, I also want you to learn to disengage; to connect and then disconnect at the end of a working day. If you don't, you 'leak' energy, and then depression and tiredness can follow. You are not meant to carry others' burdens for them at the expense of your own wellbeing. Over-sympathising and over-caring result in an overburdened carer.

During my talks I ask the audience to try the simple exercise of putting on an imaginary coat/jacket as their working uniform when caring for others, to feel that they are wearing an extra layer of protection during their working day which can absorb all the stress, upset, aggression, despair and loneliness that may be encountered. I then ask them to remove this imaginary jacket before they enter their own home at the end of the caring day, to leave it on a peg outside to be cleaned overnight, so preventing them from carrying over into their own lives the stresses and strains of those they care for. The feedback from this exercise has been very positive, for we need to understand that we do the best we can. If we have slipped up, we are human and we can always start again tomorrow – but from a place that is not overloaded with the emotional stresses of others, for our imaginary jacket leaves all that outside our home, giving us the chance to restore ourselves. If I am giving healing in hospices or talking at care homes I will always send a prayer up to ask for my protection for the day. Discover a ritual that works for you and that falls in line with your beliefs. Don't overlook this important aspect of self-preservation. You are worth it!

GUILT

Guilt can play a terrible part in disturbing our wellbeing. Feeling guilty can be a self-defeating habit which does not serve us well. Know that you deserve time alone and that, rather than feeling guilty about a situation, you will take the action that you can when you can.

I find the following prayer, known as the Serenity Prayer, extremely helpful in those situations where the pressure of looking after others can become unbearable:

God, give me the serenity to accept the things I cannot change, the courage to change the things I can, and the wisdom to know the difference.

MEDITATION

Taking time out in the form of meditation is so beneficial. Giving yourself the opportunity to sit with your emotional pain, like a mother with a child, helps dissipate anxiety, for your emotional stress is not then fighting for your attention and so escalating its force. You are making the space to pay it mindful attention. Then visualise and breathe out the discomfort.

Meditation does not require any specific beliefs, it is simply a journey of rediscovery of our inner selves. It can help keep us peaceful and positive, and it develops inner strength. I am so pleased that thousands of care staff regularly use my meditations and tell me of their benefits. The meditation in the box that follows will help you to free yourself from feeling overburdened, to maintain your boundaries, and to remember who you are outside of work, thereby helping you to see which are your stresses and what stresses of others you may be shouldering. You may choose to record it and play it back to yourself. I have made an audio recording for carers in my training pack, but reading it quietly to yourself will also have a positive effect. Find a comfy chair and a room where you will not be disturbed. This will only take a few minutes.

MEDITATION EXERCISE

Close your eyes . . . breathe, relax, feel your feet on the floor and imagine a beautiful light of protection swirling around you. You feel warm,
safe and nurtured within this light. Take a deeper breath . . . go into
the stillness, observe emerging thoughts and feelings with detachment. This is your time for you.

Let's begin . . .

Think of yourself sitting on a soft and comfortable swing seat in a
beautiful garden. There is a gentle warm breeze against your face,
and you are gently swinging back and forth in a relaxed way on your
swing seat, letting the slow rocking movements relax you as you look
over this beautiful garden. Feel the warmth of the sun and take a slow
deep breath as you savour this moment in this beautiful garden.

The colours are vibrant. You notice a shimmering butterfly as it
freely moves and hovers over the array of colourful flowers. You enjoy
the fragrances, the different textures and the play of light on the
wings of the butterfly. The place is filled with sweet aromas. Breathe
in deeply . . . listen to the birds and notice the trees as they gracefully
give way to the gentle breeze. The sky is blue, and bright. Take a
moment to enjoy what you see. Do not rush, give yourself time. There
are no clocks here, no mobile phones . . .

Stop and feel the peace. You feel happy and savour the peacefulness . . . See that placed in your lap is a beautiful cloak, it is shining
with golden light and you wrap it around you, feeling secure and com-
forted within it. Take a deep breath in and sigh out any lingering
tension. Now gently allow yourself to think back to those in your care
with compassionate detachment. And know that you have done the
best that you can for them for that day.

Breathe deeply.

Now see those in your care/family, either collectively or individually, in their own beautiful bubbles of golden light. They are happy and content within these light-shining bubbles. Very gently, and with no sense of guilt and regret, you are able to gently blow these bubbles away from you. See those in your care gently receding into the distance – they are safe, protected, and able to enjoy their own company too, leaving you shining, glowing, enjoying the peace of being within your own energy, nothing to say, do or give . . .

This is your time, time for you. Take another deep breath. Sometimes we run from ourselves and others; we are so busy, so stressed we lose the connection with our own life, our own soul . . . Breathe deeply three more times . . . Be with yourself for a few moments; feel how good, how restorative it is to be connected to yourself for even a few brief moments . . .

Now very gently, maintaining this sense of peace and connectedness, give thanks to yourself for all that you are, all that you have been and all that you will be. Know that the cloak or light of protection is there for you to put on every day before work or at other stressful times – and that the stability and comfort of feeling yourself rooted on the earth is there daily for your benefit. Know that when you allow this time to connect with yourself and know yourself, then you can truly connect with others in a deeper and more nourishing way, understanding that meditations like this one can help you prevent feeling overwhelmed.

Feel yourself very slowly coming back to the room . . . very gently move your fingers . . . your toes. . .

Welcome back.

Tools for survival!

The challenges of caring – particularly for people with dementia, who need constant reassurance, help through the mire of confusion and distress, or dealing with aggression and emotional distress – require high levels of emotional skill. To cope with high levels of demand, we need emotional support to sustain motivation, and we need recognition for the hidden tasks which can appear to be thankless. But too often we will have only ourselves to give the support and appreciation needed. So here are some personal skills to explore to help prevent burnout and to sustain you through the challenging times.

PERSONAL SKILLS

- Develop emotional strength and courage to witness and endure distress while sustaining an attitude of hope.
- Take one step at a time.
- Nurture humour.
- Be able to grieve and let go.
- Develop the ability to reflect.
- Use nature to remain inspired.
- Have self respect: value yourself, make friends with yourself again.
- Give yourself time and space for relaxation wherever possible.
- Have a thankful heart and count your blessings.
- Talk to others: banish isolation, ask for help.

BE POSITIVE

Keeping positive and maintaining a positive attitude is easier said than done. But this attitude can encourage self-belief in yourself and those you care for. Being positive brings more energy, building hope and motivating those around you to experience better relationships. Never underestimate the importance of a smile, to both the giver and the receiver, and remember smiling is infectious! In my workshops I ask participants to try an experiment with me. I ask them to think about something that has annoyed or stressed them, while smiling and raising their gaze to look upwards. It is so interesting to see how much more difficult it is to focus on negative emotions while adjusting your physical being like this.

HUMOUR PRESCRIPTION

'One day I sat thinking in despair when I felt a hand on my shoulder and a voice in my ear say, Cheer up, things could be worse. So sure enough I cheered up and things got worse!'

Humour is a wonderful tension reliever; it is no wonder that most of those in the caring industry develop quite a black sense of humour. It's a useful coping mechanism to discharge stress and the build-up of anxiety. It is vital that we discover ways that work best for us. Dr Patch Adams from the Gesundheit Institute (about whom the film *Patch Adams*, starring Robin Williams, was made) dresses up as a clown while doing his rounds. It works for him!

KEEP THE CANDLE LIT

A practice that I have found extremely helpful in keeping me balanced and sane during times of caring for others has been to imagine that a candle is within me, placed in the area of the stomach where we hold so much stress. See this candle being lit within you, emanating a warm comforting glow inside, relaxing any tension in the warmth of its gentle light. Then, every day, keep checking in with this candle: has it gone out? Do you need to relight it? If so, do so. Try to keep this candle lit during times of stress or depression; it is a simple but effective practice.

KEEPING A BALANCE

It is important that we try to maintain a good balance between giving and receiving care. In my workshops I ask participants to list how many forms of care they give in work and at home – including such small tasks as feeding the fish. I then ask them to list how many forms of care they receive: being cooked for, driven, hugged, etc. Finally, to compare the difference. So often the sheets are unbalanced, with all of us giving much more care than we are receiving. There are dangers of potential burnout when this is the case, for we are not getting nurtured and perhaps we don't realise this until it's too late. So I encourage people to look at their balance of care and to ask for support where possible to bring things back into a healthy balance. If you don't ask you don't get, and gentle reminders will not always be rejected, we just assume they will! Give others the opportunity to help you, be it friends, family or colleagues. Share out some of your chores. For it's no help you going down with the ship!

SALT WATER

If I have given healing or any kind of personal care I always wash my hands in salt water afterwards. This helps clear my energy field from that of the other person. The salt contains properties that cleanse the parts that other soaps cannot reach. It works on an energetic level, and I recommend you try it once in a while.

POETIC SOLUTIONS

I wrote the following poem during the toughest times of caring for my mother. These were words of comfort to myself when the situation seemed so hopeless. Consider writing a message or poem, or drawing a picture, as a way of rekindling your spirit and motivation. I share my poem at the end of every conference and it has become like a personal mantra to remind me to keep pushing forward during the tough times.

Planting
If you plant a seed
And it takes root elsewhere
Don't turn your back
The seed is still there
It's sowing that matters
The courage to try
Nerves may be shattered
But the seed cannot die.

Amanda Waring

REFLECTION

The ability to reflect is a useful tool where you can look over what has been challenging or difficult and consider ways by which you may be able to overcome the negative emotions or situations. Reflection can strengthen self-esteem as we learn from our mistakes, observing our feelings and building on positive experiences. Keeping a diary is a good way to reflect on our experiences. Reflect on what you enjoy most about caring for others, and keep these aspects to the fore to shore up morale.

TREAT YOURSELF

During times of stress, give yourself permission to take time for yourself: take a long hot bath, go to the movies, walk by the sea, listen to music, visit friends, go dancing, visit a museum, read a good book, have a massage, open yourself up to another world outside care. Enjoy finding out different ways to nurture yourself. Try to eat healthily to support your body. Try five minutes meditation every day to re-focus yourself.

Release stress through sound: sing or shout. A good scream can do wonders – as long as you let the neighbours know! During my darkest times I would go out into the field we have at the back of our house and, head down, belly on the ground, scream into the earth, which was cathartic and freeing. I would always thank the earth – the earth mother – for having absorbed and transmuted my pain.

NIGHT-TIME CARE

Making sure those you care for are comfortable at night is so important – but it can be very tough on the carer. It often means you will have inadequate or disturbed sleep, which can impact on the body's ability to suppress illness. Here are some tips from www.myhomelife.org.uk to help you adjust and keep healthy:

- organise your sleep time well during the day, making sure friends and family help you get the sleep you need
- eat healthy food at regular times
- limit caffeine intake
- wear loose clothing and shoes
- have regular health checks
- get as much daylight as possible when you can
- be aware you may have problems with concentration, so take extra care when driving

Keep inspired

I have gained great strength from the people I have found inspirational in my life: my heroes and heroines. Take time to think of the people *you* admire, their qualities and how those might influence your work in a positive way. I also like to do an exercise in my workshops where we explore our alter ego/superhero carer, which helps enhance our abilities to work with older people. I allow five minutes for participants to draw their own superhero/super carer and to explain their super powers to the rest of us. It is great fun. Ideas have included: my superhero has feet that never tire, legs that never ache; I have a special hat I can put on when my patience is wearing thin to rejuvenate my tolerance levels; I have earmuffs that only allow praise and not criticism to come through. Consider developing a superhero of your own, to relieve stress and refocus you on the qualities and abilities you need to help you through the tough times.

I have found quotations a powerful personal aid to keep me focused and on track when I feel stale or without purpose – a state we all can slip into when challenged.

When caring for others seems an uphill struggle, and you feel you are not actually achieving anything or making a difference, consider the following quote:

To laugh often and much; to win the respect of intelligent people and the affection of children; to earn the appreciation of honest critics and endure the betrayal of false friends; to appreciate beauty, to find the best in others; to leave the world a bit better, whether by a healthy child, a garden patch, or a redeemed social condition; to know even one life has breathed easier because you have lived. This is to have succeeded!

Ralph Waldo Emerson

My granny used to keep a commonplace book of quotations, which she would read to me every now and then. I loved the succinct, simple wisdom expressed. Here are a few of my favourite quotes that keep me motivated and inspired:

> If you can imagine it you can achieve it, if you can dream it you can become it.
>
> *William Arthur Ward*

> He can who thinks he can, he won't who thinks he can't.
>
> *Orison Swett Marden*

> Life is not measured by the number of breaths we take, but by the number of moments that take our breath away.
>
> *Anon*

> Nothing great was ever achieved without enthusiasm.
>
> *Winston Churchill*

> We are all of us spiritual beings having an earthly experience.
>
> *Stephen Covey*

Consider sharing your favourite quotes or sayings with other staff and those in your care. Every day I receive a quote or thought for the day via email from the Brahma Kumaris, the World Spiritual University, and I thought I would share a few with you:

> Whatever you are experiencing in your mind now is what you put there earlier on.

> Fill every thought with determination, every step with courage and every word with love.

When you remain stable in the truth that your original nature is peace it gives the other person an opportunity to realise their own truth.

Today dissolve each obstacle by considering it to be a gift.

ASKING FOR HELP

So often we keep silent in our pain. I know I have. We may feel ashamed that we are unable to cope a moment longer. At my conferences I ask the doctors and nurses if any of them are caring for an older relative outside of their professional capacity. More and more hands go up, and we discuss the profound challenges of caring at work and at home – where there can never be a break between the two areas, when the battle to fight off depression while feeling overwhelmed seems never-ending.

When you feel seriously out of your depth and unable to cope, where do you go, who do you call? For myself, the build-up of emotional and physical exhaustion from looking after my mother as she was dying while I was heavily pregnant with my son was unrelenting and remorseless, even though she was a wonderful patient. I couldn't cope with my grief at losing my mother coupled with the dichotomy of bringing new life into the world. At that time I would have given anything to know that my mother would live even if it meant sacrificing my own pregnancy. That, on top of caring for my aggressive alcoholic father and no sleep for days on end, tipped me over the edge. I found myself driving to the top of a steep hill with the intention of driving off it and taking my own life. In my despair I just wanted to stop the world and get off. I sped up dramatically – but as I almost reached the top there appeared in front of me, from nowhere it seemed, a small deer standing in the middle of the road. It was two in the morning. I screeched to a halt, for I realised that I couldn't kill a deer. And if I couldn't kill a deer, I couldn't kill myself or my child.

I thanked the deer, and now find that at challenging times I will see a deer in my field of vision – a reminder, perhaps. The deer stopped me in my tracks and I returned to a more rational way of thinking. I drove home and immediately phoned the Samaritans, who were wonderful.

So pick up the phone. Call someone. Don't let things get out of control as I did, trying to be a good daughter and not giving myself the care I needed. Call on your faith, your God if you have one; pray, contact those in multi-faith organisations for help, contact care support groups. The internet will provide a rich source of support groups. Don't suffer alone or see your vulnerability as a weakness. It is merely a stage that you can and will move through in time – but you need not do this alone.

Caring for the impossible

Caring for my father while he was dying was impossibly difficult due to his frightening alcoholic rages, abuse and threatening, out-of-control behaviour. We had a love-hate relationship. My mother had died a few years before and I was a single mother trying to look after my father, who lived in my village but didn't want to live with me.

In my talks I discuss what helped me in relation to caring for an impossible man, which was to see his behaviour as coming from his own pain somewhere deep within him. I could see him as a wounded animal, shouting through his unresolved emotional issues, which made it easier for me to still care for him and maintain some compassion. I remind myself that behaviour is not who the person is, it is an acting out of a fraction of that whole person, and that we all have our dark side and our light side. It depends which side we choose to feed that will dominate our behaviour. We have a choice.

We also have a choice to walk away if someone is being unbearably abusive. Which indeed was what the Macmillan doctor told me. But because Dad was falling so frequently, was incontinent and refusing any other carer but me, I felt as if I were falling between the cracks and had no options. At that time I did not have a network of friends or family to help me out of this cycle. It was only when my brother, who was working in London, told Dad that he would have to give up his work to look after him as the strain on me was too much that Dad gave in, going for some respite care at a local nursing home. However, the home had to be persuaded as they felt Dad was too aggressive. He went on probation, as it were, for a few weeks.

Dad did settle there, but I went every day and had feelings of relief and guilt and confusion. As Dad got frailer his anger lessened and he realised that I would have been unable to meet all the medical needs he now had. And I finally let go of my need to be the perfect daughter.

MAINTAINING MOMENTUM

I know it is so hard when you as a carer may be caught between the sad eyes of those you care for and the hardened gaze of those managers who are putting profits above people. Our society, bereft of self-esteem, is being suffocated by its own sense of powerlessness, and it takes a great deal of passion and foresight to lift oneself out of the collective mire of apathy. So where possible make it fun! As Emma Goldman said: 'If I can't dance, I don't want to be part of your revolution.' Feel your path as a varied, rich and uplifting experience, and ground yourself in missions of higher good and service.

I have managed to keep my momentum going as a relentless campaigner for the elderly by using aspects of my abilities as an actress, writer, healer and film director to manifest a direct connection to those in the caring industry. I believe in holding a vision of excellent care, leading by example – I love this quote by Marianne Williamson:

> We are all meant to shine as children do . . . And as we let our light shine, we unconsciously give others permission to do the same. As we are liberated from our own fear, our presence automatically liberates others.

Passion and persistence can change the world, and at my talks I hope to inspire others to work long and hard at what they believe in. I have a tremendous desire for social change, and see passion and persistence as the key to creating this.

In my workshops I love to quote the following story about Sir Winston Churchill who, at the age of eighty, was asked to address the Oxford Student Union. He stood on the stage and said: 'Never give up.' There was a thirty-second pause as he looked the students in the eyes before saying again, 'Never give up.' Another minute passed as he looked them more deeply in the eyes, and then finally said: 'Never give up.' And with that he left the stage. Perfect!

I have been blessed to make personal friendships with those people who hold the same vision I do, including Dr Patch Adams from the Gesundheit Institute; Dadi Janki, spiritual leader of Brahma Kumaris; and David Sheard from Dementia Matters. If I have lost my focus or drive, their work refreshes my spirits and inspires me to find the joy in service. So find your own inspirers and co-travellers who can lift your spirits and keep your feet on the path.

I believe that sacrifice, responsibility and struggle are horrible ways in which to motivate yourself. You will start to blame or resent the very thing you are passionate about. Instead, define success as something achievable, so that you don't feel overwhelmed. I define my own success as something like this: Did I try? Did I give my time? Did I never give up?

Do not try to put success in things or outcomes but more in the process of the journey you are creating in the work you do. Don't ever sacrifice your need to be creative. Creativity is one of the best medicines; it is essential nourishment and can be the very soul of our sense of self-worth.

ANXIOUS BUTTERFLIES

There will always be times when the going gets tough. When I felt overwhelmed with anxiety before appearing as an actress in shows, suffering unbearable nervous butterflies in my stomach, my granny used to say to me: 'You can't avoid the butterflies – but the trick is to get them to fly in formation!' And that's what I would do.

We can rarely avoid stress. We just have to get better at living alongside it and keep on keeping on!

～

'From caring comes courage.'
Lao Tzu

CHAPTER 9

Honouring and Celebrating
Our Elders

Honouring and celebrating our elders is a vital factor at the heart of care. An older person's life experiences may give clues to their current behaviour and emotional response to circumstances. Elders very often have the wisdom of experience and a wider perspective, helping us tackle our own insecurities.

This chapter contains a variety of activities and information from my 'What do you see?' training pack. These celebrate intergenerational idiosyncrasies, bringing the generations and the wider community together and honouring, celebrating and utilising the life experiences of those in your care to enrich both your and their experience.

Honour me

I am often asked to go into care homes to not only train the staff around dignity in care and person-centred care but, wearing my performer's hat, to also entertain the residents and relatives and talk about the work I do and the importance of care that honours and celebrates.

There will often be some elders too poorly to come down for this so I always ask, if it is appropriate and acceptable to them, to visit them in their rooms and share a little of what I am doing downstairs to help them feel included. This has often resulted in my singing lullabies to those who are dying, holding their hands, stroking their hair, telling them that they have touched so many others' lives and that I honour all that they have experienced, shared and loved till now. These private quiet moments remind me of our profound need for gratitude, the need to be acknowledged, the need to be remembered.

When I am downstairs with the relatives and residents I use my drum, having been trained in Native American traditions, to softly play like a heartbeat over each individual where this ritual of recognising the life of an elder begins. I tell them that their life has been worthwhile, that they represent seven generations forward and seven generations back, and that the echo of the drum honours and recognises the journey of their family and themselves till this point in time, celebrating all that they are, all that they have been and all that they will be.

I love seeing the mixed response of tears, surprise, relief, peace and laughter, the soul healing that comes when someone takes the time to honour and celebrate the life of another.

Celebrating history

It is important to be able to discuss points of interest in shared memories as part of the living history of an elder person, to be able to explore and celebrate individual life experiences and to tap into an elder's knowledge as a history keeper. As an exercise in your care setting, see how far back individuals have memories of historical events. There is a rich vein of experiences that can provide topics of conversation for everyone, as well as opportunities for staff and relatives to learn! You could make it like a fun history test: 'I was there when . . .'

SIGNIFICANT EVENTS CHECKLIST

Here are some significant dates from my 'What do you see?' training pack. They will tell you a little about the type of events residents will be familiar with. They can be used to help you find out about their lives; public events can be a memory jogger or a prompt for general conversation. They can also be used to develop activities.

I have left the last several years for you to add and contribute to, through your own memories and the memories of your family members.

Childhood
1920s

1921   Marie Stopes opened the first family planning clinic in London

1922   Ford sold a million Model Ts – the first 'cheap' mass-produced car

The British Broadcasting Company (BBC) was formed to broadcast the first regular wireless programmes in Britain

1923   The Irish Civil War ended

The first Wembley Cup Final held

1926   The General Strike

1927   The first 'talkies' (films with sound) appeared – the very first was *The Jazz Singer*

Charles Lindbergh made the first solo non-stop flight across the Atlantic

1928   Alexander Fleming discovered penicillin

Women over 21 years of age allowed to vote

1929   The Wall Street Crash of New York's stock market started the Great Depression

The Labour Party became the largest political party in Britain for the first time

Youth
1930s

1930   Amy Johnson flew solo from London to Australia

1930s   The Great Depression

1932   BBC's TV public service began

1933   The first female announcer employed by the BBC

Adolf Hitler became the German Chancellor

1934   Fred Perry won the men's tennis championship at Wimbledon

'Cat's eyes' (reflecting road studs) invented

1935   Silver Jubilee of King George V and Queen Mary

Mickey Mouse appeared in colour for the first time

1936   King George V died and was succeeded by his son, Edward VIII, on 20 January

Edward VIII abdicated on 10 December to marry Mrs Wallis Simpson (an American divorcee); thereafter they were known as the Duke and Duchess of Windsor. He was succeeded by his brother, the Duke of York – King George VI

Crystal Palace destroyed by fire

Billy Butlin opened his first holiday camp at Skegness

The Jarrow March began on 5 October

1937   Coronation of King George VI and Queen Elizabeth on
        12 May

        Neville Chamberlain succeeded Stanley Baldwin as
        Prime Minister

1938   Two-thirds of homes wired for electricity from new
        National Grid

        Nylon produced for the first time

        The Beano comic launched

1939   Britain declared war on Germany on 3 September

Young adult years
1940s

1940   Winston Churchill became Prime Minister

        Dunkirk evacuation

        Battle of Britain

        The Blitz began on 7 September

1941   Japan attacked US Navy at Pearl Harbor in Hawaii on
        7 December – America joined the Allies

        Women without children called up to help with the
        war effort

1944   D Day – Allies started invasion of France on 6 June

1945   VE Day – Victory in Europe Day after Germany's
        unconditional surrender on 8 May

        Atom bomb dropped on Hiroshima on 6 August

        VJ Day, 15 August

        Labour Government elected in July

1946   The first family allowances paid – 5 shillings per child
        per week for second and subsequent children

1947   India became an independent State, leaving the British Empire

Christian Dior launched the 'New Look'

Princess Elizabeth and Lieutenant Philip Mountbatten married on 20 November

1948   Formation of the National Health Service (NHS)

The Berlin blockade and airlift

Prince Charles born on 14 November

Long-playing (LP) records were invented

Adulthood
1950s and 60s

1950   Princess Anne born on 15 August

1951   The Archers serial started on the radio, 1 January

The Festival of Britain took place

Guy Burgess and Donald Maclean defected to Russia

1952   King George VI died, 6 February

First commercial jet airliner, the Comet, began service with BOAC on 2 May

Last of the old trams ran in London

1953   Everest conquered on 29 May

Coronation of Queen Elizabeth II on 2 June – event was televised; many families bought televisions

1954   Food rationing ended

Roger Bannister ran the first 4-minute mile

1955   Commercial television introduced in Britain

Rock 'n' roll music hit Britain as Bill Haley and the Comets went to No 1 with 'Rock Around the Clock'

James Dean killed, 30 September

Princess Margaret decided not to marry Group Captain Peter Townsend

1956   Britain's first nuclear power station opened at Calder Hall on 17 October

1958   Munich air disaster – eight Manchester United football players killed, 6 February

1959   First major motorway opened – the M1 – on 2 November

1961   Berlin Wall built

Contraceptive pill became available for married women only

1962   Cuban missile crisis

James Hanratty hanged for the A6 murder, 4 April

'Love Me Do' became first hit for Beatles, 5 October

1963   Profumo affair

Kim Philby defected to the Soviet Union

President John F Kennedy assassinated on 22 November

1966   England's football team beat Germany in the World Cup Final at Wembley

144 killed in Aberfan disaster, 21 October

Ian Brady and Myra Hindley jailed for life for the Moors Murders, 6 May

1968   The Abortion Act of 1967 came into effect, 27 April

1969   Moon landing, 20 July

Mature years
1970s

1970   Equal Pay Act passed so that women got 'the same pay for the same work'

1971   Britain introduced decimal currency on 15 February

1972   Miners went on all-out strike, 9 January

       'Bloody Sunday' in Londonderry, 30 January

1973   Britain joined the European Economic Community, 1 January

1974   Year of IRA bombings

1975   Sex Discrimination Act passed to give women greater opportunity of equality in the workplace

1976   Race Relations Act passed, making it illegal to discriminate on grounds of race in housing, employment and education

1978   The world's first test-tube baby born, 25 July

1979   Conservative Party elected and Margaret Thatcher became Britain's first female Prime Minister

       Number of days lost through strike action exceeded those in General Strike year of 1926

       Earl Mountbatten assassinated by the IRA, 27 August

Retirement
1980s onwards

1981   Prince Charles and Lady Diana Spencer married in St Paul's Cathedral, 29 July

       Race riots in Brixton, Toxteth and Moss Side

1982   Britain at war with Argentina in the Falkland islands

       Prince William born on 21 June

1983   Cruise missiles installed at Greenham Common

        Breakfast television began broadcasting

1984   National Union of Mine Workers called national strike
        against pit closures
        Conservative party Brighton bombing by IRA,
        12 October

1985   First government-promoted public education campaign
        about risk of AIDS

1987   Zeebrugge ferry disaster, 6 March

        October: great storm swept across southeast England –
        15 million trees felled

1988   Lockerbie bombing, 21 December

        Hillsborough football disaster; 96 Liverpool fans died,
        15 April

        Berlin Wall came down, 9 November

1990   Poll tax riots took place in London

        Mrs Thatcher resigned as leader of Conservative Party –
        replaced by John Major

        Nelson Mandela freed

1991   Britain took part in the Gulf War against Iraq

        War started in Yugoslavia

1992   Princess Royal granted divorce from Captain Mark
        Phillips

        Part of Windsor Castle destroyed by fire

1994   Channel Tunnel opened

1996   Prince Charles and Princess Diana divorced

1997   'New Labour' Party elected in May – Tony Blair
        became Prime Minister

Hong Kong returned to Chinese rule on 1 July

Diana, Princess of Wales, killed in Paris on 31 August; Mother Theresa died later in the same week

The Queen and Prince Philip celebrated their golden wedding on 20 November

1998   Easter Peace Agreement in Northern Ireland

1999   Bill Clinton, the US President, in impeachment trial – found 'not guilty'

Prince Edward married Sophie Rhys-Jones, 19 June

2000   Prince William celebrated his 18th birthday

Anti-capitalist May Day riots in London and other major cities around the world

2001   9 September: the Twin Towers of the World Trade Center in New York bombed

2002   Princess Margaret and Queen Elizabeth the Queen Mother died within weeks of each other, just before the Queen celebrated her Golden Jubilee by touring across the UK and the world

Princess Anne celebrated her 50th birthday

2003   50th anniversary of the Coronation

The war in Iraq began

England won the Rugby World Cup

Wayne Rooney EU footballer of the year

Concorde flew its last commercial flight

2004   Indian Ocean tsunami disaster

Celebrate me

Think about what ways you or your organisation can celebrate the life experience and wisdom of the elders you care for.

I suggest creating a wisdom/advice book that collates and records the thoughts and stories of those in your care, which can then be shared. Or you can use multimedia creatively and make short films of the lives of others to be shared with relatives.

REMINISCENCE

Reminiscence work can be beneficial to create links between the past and the present and to reinforce an elder's sense of self-worth and individual identity. Reminiscence work can be an empowering activity and can result in carers learning new information about residents. Use multi-sensory prompts such as music, objects and artefacts. Themes can include childhood, schooldays, family life, evenings out, adjusting to life after the war, rationing, etc.

Using the list below, explore ways you could introduce music, poetry, a creative activity (craft or drama), a story or poem or song to illustrate and celebrate some memories of those in your care. Build up a kit to use during group sessions.

My best outfit
Individuals might like to draw the favourite smart clothes they remember, or you could draw for them from their descriptions. Include as many details as possible.

Touching textiles
Gather some items of different textures, for example a velvet dress, soft kid gloves, silk stockings, fur wrap, stiff starched collar. Encourage each individual to touch the items, especially those who have difficulty speaking. Those who can talk can describe how the objects feel and remember if they wore similar things.

Smelling scents

Give everyone in the group the opportunity to smell a fragrance. People could then shut their eyes and try to remember and describe a favourite scent they used to wear.

Make-up

If a conversation about make-up has come up, some individuals might want to try on modern make-up. Of course others in the group might not want to do this at all!

Getting ready to go out

Ask people to think back to when they used to get ready to go out for a special evening. Ask them to describe what they did, from washing their hair to putting on make-up or Brylcreem. Discuss what young people wear now when they go out, using pictures from contemporary magazines or asking about younger relatives. Compare the differences and similarities with their youth.

Music

Listen to CDs together, if you feel the period is appropriate. Ask about the memories the music evokes.

A night at the flicks

Group members might like to make a scrapbook of films and film stars, using postcards and pictures from magazines and books. If people express an interest in seeing a particular film again, you could arrange a viewing. You could even provide food people remember eating at the cinema such as popcorn and ice cream.

Intergenerational differences

The intergenerational 'then and now' tables that follow provide general comparisons that can help staff of different ages and backgrounds to familiarise themselves with the social backdrop to daily life as it used to be when today's 85-year-olds were growing up. Use them to enjoy building a deeper connection through discussion with those in your care — for instance, which aspects of life do you consider better then or now, and why?

Society's trends and values

Today's culture	Former culture
Little sense of common purpose	There was a more common sense of purpose, particularly during the war years when people tended to pull together and help each other out, even strangers
'Me culture' with personal branding	Brands were not available to the masses as they are today
Individualism rules	Interdependence and the 'greater good' was taught in schools until the late 70s
People are less embarrassed or reluctant to go to the state for help. Strong welfare state culture going back two or more generations	People did not want to rely on anyone else and there was a sense of pride about not needing 'welfare' or handouts. Before 1948 there was no welfare state; there were workhouses for the destitute
There is now a 'blame' culture	Generally speaking people were expected to be responsible for their own actions and it was not considered acceptable to 'pass the buck'. If a person tripped on a pavement they would not dream of blaming the council
Privacy and individualism are the norm. There is a different kind of community spirit; less personal responsibility for community	People enjoyed public communal activities such as going to church or a community facility. The community was valued and generally this centred around location

Today's culture	Former culture
Youth culture; 'teenagers' have been a recognised stratum of society since the 1950s	No youth culture. Mothers and daughters, fathers and sons dressed the same, and teenagers were not heard of – you were either a child or a 'grown up'
Flexible roles between men and women	Gender roles were much more clearly defined
Class status is less clearly defined and there is more 'meritocracy' between classes; status based on ability fuels aspiration. Reverse snobbery is now more fashionable, as middle classes 'dumb themselves down' to become transparent in a 'classless society'	Class status was more clearly defined and fixed. Working classes aspired to the middle class and the middle class to the upper class. There were three distinguishable groups within the middle class, often easy to identify. People aspired to speak the 'Queens English' or 'BBC English'
People today are less concerned about what the neighbours might think – many do not know their neighbours and therefore may be less sensitive or considerate as relationships are more remote	Community spirit was strong as people moved around less and knew their neighbours. People were concerned what the neighbours thought ('keeping up appearances') – this meant people were unlikely to 'make a scene' or upset their neighbours
Feelings are discussed openly – we are emotionally literate	Feelings were discussed less – 'stiff upper lip'; it was not considered good to show too much emotion
There is a lack of generosity and common courtesy towards the public – people talk less in the street to strangers, there is a sense of distrust towards them	People in the street acknowledged each other when passing by, doffing a hat or greeting 'Good morning' etc. Strangers may have been treated with suspicion but were still acknowledged as people
People work long hours but doing the minimum is acceptable in some workplaces. People change jobs frequently	There was a strong work ethic – diligence and hard work valued; going the extra mile appreciated and promoted. People tended to stay in one job for a long time

General lifestyle

Now	Then
Life in the fast lane: speed of living faster	Pace of life was slower; more time to talk over the fence to a neighbour
Materialistic, consumerist society – extravagant lifestyles more mainstream; throwaway habit has led to inability to get things mended	Many people had less, and if they had it, it was considered bad taste to show it. It was a 'make do and mend' society in which people were encouraged to make things last. There was less emphasis on having to buy the latest gadgets
New things are valued	A sense of continuity was valued – the old sweater with holes in it was preserved; traditions such as 'penny for the Guy' on Bonfire Night were upheld
Shopping is now a leisure activity with chain stores and supermarkets providing huge choice	Shopping was a necessity for most people and there was far less to choose from
Food from all over the world is available and enjoyed	Preferred food was plain cooking: 'meat and two veg'; roast beef and Yorkshire pudding; steamed puddings. 'High tea' would be smoked haddock or sardines on toast with bread and butter and cakes, scones and plenty of tea
Both tea and coffee are enjoyed	'A nice cup of tea' was a socially acceptable drink, with accompanying brewing rituals
Drinking at a local pub is enjoyed equally by men and women	Having a pint in a local pub was much more a male activity than a female one
Easy credit means that many people have the opportunity of buying things before they can afford it	Credit was not available and the culture was one of saving up for something before you could think about buying it

Now	Then
Global transport – cheap flights have opened up travel to the masses	Most people stayed in the UK for holidays, if they were lucky enough to have one. A much smaller population of the better off travelled abroad, unless it was for the armed forces
Respect for the Royal family and authority in general has lessened	Most of the country respected and held the Royal family and authority in general in high regard
Holidays linked to Christian festivals have less prominence	As a Christian country most people, even the non-believers, knew the true meaning of festivals such as Christmas, Easter and Whitsun
Christianity and its way of life now marginalised and valued at the level of other religions. It is not taught as the central focus of our culture in schools any more. Forty-five per cent of people feel Christianity has been marginalised. Secular multi-culturalism and 'politically correct' local government policies	Christianity was the bedrock of western civilisation, underpinning the state and the provision of education, hospitals, charity, legal and political institutions. The Judeo-Christian heritage was a great influence
'Pick and mix' lifestyle	There was a more specific and rigid set of rules and expectations
Work ethic is less puritanical. There is now a National Lottery and gambling is more acceptable. Money is celebrated and flaunted. People feel they must buy the latest model of car, kitchen or gadget to keep up appearances, encouraged by aggressive advertising and marketing	Puritanism still influenced public behaviour and the work ethic did not encourage extravagance or 'flashing money around'. Advertising and marketing were softer and less aggressive. There was less emphasis on buying new things and goods were made to last longer

Continued ➤

Now	Then
Boasting about achievements and self-promotion are now more commonplace and acceptable. People admire those who make a lot of money	Boasting of any kind was frowned upon; 'selling yourself' was not seen as a virtue in today's sense. There was more attention to the greater good than self-gratification, and acts of charity and kindness for others were held in high regard. Humility, modesty and understatement were highly valued

Family life

Now	Then
Marriage is now a lifestyle option among a range of other possibilities from co-habitation to same-sex unions – traditional role of marriage less important	Marriage was central to family life –there was a common understanding about what this meant, protected by government policy and the legal system. It was considered shameful to have children out of wedlock or to be divorced
Nuclear family is the norm	Extended families lived within closer range of each other until people started taking jobs out of their area
Mothers are more in charge	Fathers ruled and were seen as head of the house and family – the mother was usually at home with the children. Fewer women worked when they had young children
Home-making has been commercialised – fewer women have the time for such activities, which now have to be fitted around work	Home-making skills were valued: housekeeping, sewing, cooking. Most women gained their self-esteem from these activities and felt judged on how clean, fresh and well maintained their house was

Now	Then
Days of the week not distinguished much	More distinguishing between the days of the week and their associations – Monday was wash day, some had fish on a Friday and many people dressed up on Sundays for going to church.
Most couples work and sometimes women are the primary breadwinners or bring in equal income from a greater selection of jobs	Men were the primary breadwinners. Most women who worked were in lower paid jobs and salaries were seen as secondary to the husband's. Some men were proud that their wives were not working
Society is more aware of rights of children	Children were not the centre of attention; adults ruled and 'grown ups' were generally looked up to.
Children eat out more with friends and family	It was not common for a child to eat out
Many meals are eaten individually as people live increasingly separate or busy lives	Family meals were a ritual. There were common rituals like saying grace or giving thanks before meals, or waiting for others to pick up a knife and fork before starting to eat
Having a shower rather than a bath is much more common	Hardly anyone had showers in their home
Friends and colleagues are valued as much as or even more than some family members	Family ties were highly valued and came before friends. Family life was sacred
Few women of working age today are involved with charity work	Women staying at home were likely to be involved in charity or voluntary work

Manners

Now	Then
Little deference towards and less respect for older people. Today there is less contact across the generations	There was more deference to older people. Children were taught to show courtesy, such as helping an old lady across the road or giving up a seat on a bus
Little modesty in dress; children wear adultstyle clothing	Modesty was a virtue, and 'nice girls' were expected to cover up and not show too much flesh
People have little shyness about showing affection in public places	Physical displays of affection in public were not considered polite
Greetings are less formal and children are more likely to call adults by their Christian names. Men and women have adopted the continental greeting of kissing each other's cheek	Greetings usually involved shaking a person's hand and saying 'How do you do?' In public, people tried not to touch strangers. When men wore hats they might lift their hat as a sign of respect, known as doffing the hat or cap
Politeness and courtesy are still valued but are becoming less common in public life	Politeness and courtesy were highly valued, and expressed in such things as holding doors open for others, walking on the right side of a lady, giving up seats to women and older people on public transport
There is greater acceptance of public assertiveness and 'making a scene'	People rarely made a scene in public and did not want to 'make a fuss'

TALKING ABOUT MY GENERATION

William James said: 'The greatest discovery of my generation is that a human being can alter his life by altering his attitudes to it.'

Let the topics in the 'then and now' table inspire you to involve younger people in the care home or with those you care for, to exchange ideas about each other's lives. In the care homes I visit I encourage staff to involve a local school. The relationship between young and old is so important; both can enrich and inspire the other. The fresh energy of children in a care home can resonate positively for a long while after any visit. Do not overlook the power of intergenerational healing.

'Look to the old, they are worthy of old age; they have seen their days and proven themselves. At this age the old can predict or give knowledge or wisdom, whatever it is.'

Black Elk, Oglala Sioux

CHAPTER 10

Creativity and
Activity in Care

'It is neither wealth nor splendor, but tranquility and occupation which give happiness.'

Thomas Jefferson

'Age should be not seen as an illness but a time of growth.'

Betty Friedan

Giving voice to our unique creativity provides us with freedom of expression and a sense of purpose that makes us feel alive. It can be as simple as arranging some flowers or our hair, or even laying a table. But it provides us with a sense of purpose and delight.

We all need a variety of activities in our lives, from daily living tasks to well-established hobbies, to give us a sense of achievement. But be mindful that, with older people, matching skills and abilities with the demands of the task in hand will ensure that the activity is not so easy as to become boring or so demanding as to become stressful.

Restoring a sense of purpose

Hope and intimacy needs can be met if elders are helped to find new companionship and are supported to overcome the feeling of dependency. Being able to continue to contribute, to share with others, to give and to receive love, help people to find peace and dignity in old age. Having a sense of purpose, and ideally of achievement, is necessary for people to continue to thrive spiritually, emotionally and physically.

The body and the mind need a level of challenge to keep them in good order. Sensitive understanding of these needs and words of encouragement can help to reduce stress and develop a sense of control, joy and wellbeing. Many older people can feel disconnected from significant people and routines, from their family or familiar surroundings. Activities such as art, music, walking or gardening can restore interest and perhaps provide new opportunities for building new relationships.

TAKING THE RIGHT STEPS

So let us help those in our care to wear their age not as a burden but as a crown. For some, being encouraged in small ways to participate using their remaining abilities can also bring real restoration of hope and belief in the 'art of the possible' in the face of illness or multiple losses. The latter are often accompanied by a lack of confidence, so it is important to ask the right questions and find out what small thing they would like to achieve or do for themselves.

SOMETHING TO AIM FOR

Having a goal to aim for is one way to motivate people. Consider using score cards, reward stickers, commitment cards to monitor progress. Sharing and keeping an eye on each other's goals can be motivating, too. Share your own goals with the people in your care so that you can support each other and deepen your relationship. Enjoy the process!

But always remember that goals must be achievable and realistic to be effective.

KEEP MOVING

Sitting for long periods can hasten physical decline. It is important to provide opportunities for people to keep active, even if it is only in small ways. Lack of sufficient physical activity has a major impact on physical and psychological health. Increasing movement and function involves a combination of motivation, self-belief and encouragement with the right level of assistance.

Exercise is particularly important as we get older. Physical activity has a positive effect on both our mood and mental agility. Maximising physical activity may even delay the onset of some illnesses and diseases of old age and prevent depression, aches and pains, sleep disorders and memory difficulties. It provides an opportunity to have fun and make new friends. Specific exercise to increase strength, flexibility and balance can rejuvenate our bodies by up to twenty years, so staying active provides the strength and power to stay independent.

THANK YOU, DOUGLAS!

'The longer you survive, the more you rely on yourself. But I had a leg amputated, so I had to come into this place. I thought, well, I've still got one leg. So I pushed myself around in my wheelchair with my foot. But they still couldn't stop trying to help – shoving me from one place to another when

I was doing all right on my own. Lots of bright smiles, but they just weren't listening.

'Then I blew my top and I told one of them where she could get off. I told her if Douglas Bader could fly a Spitfire with no legs, I could push a wheelchair with one. But she listened. And do you know, I've never had any trouble with the nurses since. They're not a bad crowd really, once they listen.

'It takes a long time to get to supper, but it works up an appetite.

'Thank you, Douglas!'

Wheelchair user in a care home

PHYSICAL AND PSYCHOLOGICAL RESULTS OF INACTIVITY

It is important to encourage and maximise every opportunity for people to move as much as possible. This can be encouraged by simple walks and talks, competitive physical games, and a range of individual and group activity choices.

The list below spells out the possible effects of inactivity – in case you need prompting to keep yourself active as well as those you care for!

Physical results of inactivity
Muscles waste and joints contract; bone changes, resulting in increased risk of fracture and long healing times; increased risk of heart and respiratory problems; reduced appetite; continence difficulties; sleep disturbance.

Psychological results of inactivity
Decreased alertness and concentration; increased impatience, irritability and hostility; increased tension, anxiety, agitation, depression; increased lethargy; decreased problem-solving ability; confusion and disorientation.

'MOVING MORE OFTEN'

The 2005 'Moving More Often' initiative of the British Heart Foundation (www.idea.gov.uk), designed for frailer older people, provides a range of activities that encourage physical activity and meet many other needs, such as improving people's self-esteem.

TAKING A ROLE

People also need roles in life to give them a sense of purpose. It is important to encourage people to still contribute wherever they can.

The following quote is from a care home resident:

'It's quite difficult not having anyone relying on you any more. I couldn't even sleep properly; I was itching to be up and doing. Even the sound of the morning shift arriving at the front door could wake me up, and they don't make much noise. Then I thought, they need a commissionaire! So that's what I do. I get up early enough to stay by the front door and let them in; then I see the night staff out. It gives me something to do – and I hope it helps them a bit. I can sleep a lot better as well.'

ROLE-PLAYING EXERCISE

Think of all the roles you play in life. They can include such roles as mother, wife, carer, grandparent, volunteer, student, church member. Now think about the elders you work with. Write down their different roles. How can we build meaningful roles into their lives? Think of ways you can encourage people to take on different roles that will provide meaning and purpose to their day within the care setting.

For example, these roles could include: gardener, lecturer/teacher, mentor, grandparent, buddy role for new residents, agony aunt/uncle, activity organiser, entertainer, cook, secretary, housekeeper.

CREATIVE AND ACTIVE CARE

Key principles to remember when exploring creativity and activity in care are:

- Older people are uniquely different, and their interests and capabilities will vary.
- You should constantly think of ways to bring people together to create a sense of community.
- Activities have health benefits, raising mood, calming or energising and preventing dependency.
- It is important that all staff use opportunities to interact with and talk to residents – and the more they know about residents the easier this is.
- It is not just about entertainment but about providing positive engagement, interest and enjoyment.

To enable you to be as effective as possible, follow these guidelines:

- Find out as much as possible about the lives of those in your care and what motivates them.
- Build up a relationship with residents and assess what they are able to do and what adaptations need to be made.

- Consider what individuals need to maximise their physical, social, emotional, sensory, spiritual, creative and mental health. Find out what they like and why they like it.
- Adapt communication methods to individual needs.
- Pay attention to choice and consent, and seek advice if unsure.
- People sometimes like to do things with others and sometimes on their own, so plan both group and individual activities. Encourage links between people to help form relationships.
- Make an activity plan with residents, with realistic and achievable aims based on interests and needs.
- Plan ahead, but be flexible and use themes that are topical or that interest residents.
- Always have a back-up plan, and review, revise and refresh regularly.
- Don't forget to include the simple domestic, everyday activities.
- Remember that older people can still learn new things.
- Analyse new activities and think how they can be adapted.
- Evaluate activities regularly against aims and objectives.
- Encourage residents, staff and relatives to be involved in planning and reviewing activities in the home.
- Keep up-to-date records.
- Include elements of surprise and novelty.
- Keep activities age and 'stage' appropriate.
- Report significant health changes or observations to relevant staff.
- Work closely with manager, team leaders and key workers and families.
- Think 'failure free', and reinforce capabilities and achievements – making a positive emotional connection is more important than the end product.

- Keep spirit, mind and body active by providing a purposeful and engaging range of activities pitched at different needs and interests.
- Remember that the wrong activity, or not enough to do, has damaging effects on health and wellbeing.
- Try to find out what people can offer and use their talents.
- Celebrate life and living together with residents, using touch, eye contact and humour.

(Compiled by Rosemary Hurtley, including material from T. Perrin (ed), 2004, The New Culture of Therapeutic Activity, Speechmark, Oxon, and R. Hurtley and J. Wenborn, The Successful Activity Co-ordinator, Age Concern, 2005.)

Motivation

Think about your own preferences for activities that are: fun; energetic; peaceful and gentle; solitary; mentally stimulating and challenging; completely new to you. Ask other staff and residents the same. It is good to hear of others' hobbies and activities; they may well inspire us to try something different for ourselves and those we care for.

Now think of activities you could try with residents under the following headings:

Stimulating the mind
Encouraging communication
Enjoying music and culture
Encouraging movement and exercise
Fun recreation/relaxation
Everyday activities
Remembering how things used to be
Working with the senses/sensory activities
Social activity
Spiritual activities

MORNING OR EVENING PERSON?

What time of the day is the best for you? Are you a morning or evening person? Do you know the best time for activities for those you care for? Finding this important factor out will allow you to adjust activities accordingly, as differing energy levels in the day will affect what people are able or want to do.

SPICE OF LIFE

Purposeful activity is not only the spice of life but essential for our mental, physical and spiritual wellbeing. There are many different types of activities which can be planned or sponta-neous. These might include: art, creative or music sessions; different types of games; social events; reminiscence groups; exercise sessions; outings; special events or themed days.

There are many opportunities for activities that are cost free and can happen spontaneously in your everyday care of an older person. They can include commenting on a newspaper or news topic; chatting with residents whilst serving tea; accompanying a resident on a walk; 'working together' to do daily household tasks such as laying tables, sorting cutlery, pairing socks, dusting, going to choose a book from the library or visiting the local shops. Enjoy them and make the most of them.

Have a range of objects and materials out on a table for people to pick up and engage in such as large print books, magazines, interesting objects to look at, puzzles or 'rummage boxes' filled with objects and memorabilia from the past.

But never forget that some residents will like to do things on their own: reading, listening to favourite music, watching a favourite programme, or just sitting quietly.

SOMETHING NEW!

Creating spontaneous and unexpected happenings becomes a great talking point for relatives, staff and residents. One care home manager arranged for a drag artist to come and perform at her home over lunchtime and that had quite an impact! But the novelty factor soon wore off as it became a regular occurrence – and it was then stopped due to residents complaining! So tread lightly when bringing new events/happenings into the care home; ask the residents and staff for their ideas.

I have listed some creative, fun, whacky activity ideas for your care setting and those you care for, to inspire you to think out of the box and unleash creative possibilities. Share any hidden talents you may have that would be appreciated in the home and that you could perhaps demonstrate or teach. Consider what activity you might introduce to enhance the quality of life for those in your care.

- A 'Desert Island Discs' day at your home where staff and residents get to play their favourite music and say what memories and associations it has for them.
- Ask older people for their favourite quotes, write them on cards and put them up around the care setting.
- Try holding some of the following workshops: singing or drumming; life drawing; magic – learning magic tricks can help with agility of mind and body, and the result of entertaining others is another reward; beauty or 'colour me beautiful'; poetry; healing and massage; shadow puppetry.
- Hold a quiz night, or start a literary appreciation/book club or film club.
- Have a chocolate tasting or wine tasting session.
- Have debate cards or moral issue cards as a fun lunchtime discussion activity.

- Start up a newsletter with the residents and relatives.
- Keep a wisdom or humour book for residents and staff to record anecdotes, quotations and personal memories they wish to share.
- Try a comedy stand-up session.

General activity ideas

Stimulating the mind (different challenges for different abilities)	Word games – anagrams, crosswords, hangman, word target, word chains; quizzes – general knowledge/current affairs related to both national and local area; commercially available kits/games – dominoes, picture matching (pelmanism); debates; newspaper discussions; memory games, e.g. Kim's Game; talking through an activity sequence, e.g. putting on a tie, tea-making; completing proverbs; jigsaw puzzles made from a favourite picture/subject; bridge or bingo (depending on ability and interest)
Encouraging communication	Discussions; drama – mime, story-making, reminiscence; reading and writing; social activities; involved in all care activities
Expressing creativity	Art – marbling, printing, silk and glass painting; crafts – candle making, needlecrafts, pottery, salt-dough modelling, wax rubbing, weaving, simple woodwork; creative writing, poetry and stories, life histories; IT using pictures and clip art; photography; dance; drama
Enjoying music and culture	Reminiscence; theme-based quizzes; games/painting to music; music appreciation; music making; singing; recitals; poetry reading; enjoying stories/plays on CD or read aloud; intergenerational projects
Encouraging movement and exercise	Ball games; balloons, batons and scarves; carpet bowls; soft darts; hockey; hoop-la; parachute games; skittles; seated exercises; singing songs and hymns together; walks and talks; quoits, skittles

Fun, relaxation, recreation and everyday activity	Cookery; gardening; pets; reading; woodwork; singing; 'rummage' boxes filled with objects and memorabilia; poetry reading/recitation; dressing up; looking at large picture books/colourful picture magazines; conversation starters – bring in some soft toys/dolls, interesting objects to pass round, to jog memories or stimulate conversation; listening to old favourites; visits with children/pets; pub-type games
Enjoying culture/special events	Variety of discussions with examples – poetry, theatre, music, art; slide shows; talks about travel, hobbies and topics of interest
Remembering how things used to be	Discussions, using props; outings; link with local libraries and schools – intergenerational projects with young people; singing
Working with the five senses	'Smelly' and 'feely' quizzes; pets brought in; cooking; herbs; flowers; pictures; listening to sounds/music; passing round interesting textured fabrics or clothes
Enjoying social interaction	Group activities such as games, quizzes, outings, tea dances and parties, group singing, table-top games; bring in some special food; sherry mornings with all the trimmings; wine/tea tastings; singing or enjoying music together
Meeting spiritual and religious needs	Singing spiritual songs and hymns; short meditations or readings; short services

(*Adapted from* The Successful Activity Co-ordinator *by Rosemary Hurtley and Jennifer Wenborn, Age Concern Books, 2005*)

The Active Care Challenge

In my training sessions and workshops I always encourage concrete consolidation of future actions in the form of written action plans or charters as a way of achieving, maintaining and improving future care.

ACTION PLAN AND CHARTER EXERCISE

Make an action plan to develop activities further with the support of management, staff, relatives and residents. Develop a charter which provides answers to the questions below:

What do we do now about the range and balance of activities in our care setting?
Where do we want to be in six months' time?
How are we going to get there?
Who will we involve? (consider possibilities both inside and outside the home; list resources outside in the wider community we can involve to help us)
Who is responsible for different aspects of the plan?

MAKING THE CHALLENGE HAPPEN

This is everybody's business, so add to the list you made in the exercise above the people not yet considered, for example the maintenance man, the laundry person, the chef, the gardener, the administrative staff. Outside the home, consider the University of the Third Age, local museums, clubs, societies, churches, schools, libraries. Each one can think of different ways they can be involved directly with residents and how they can engage and interact more. Try to *involve* and encourage people to use their abilities and not let speed or time prevent them helping and contributing in some way. Plan with older people the type of projects they might like to engage in, or make, or teach. Provide opportunities for the elders to share their skills to enrich our lives.

I hope you enjoy the process of putting creativity and

activity at the heart of your care. Remember that activities can provide meaning and purpose for everyone, including staff and relatives.

'Imagination is the magnet that pulls knowledge forward, whereas knowledge is simply our best guess at the time ... Only when you add imagination to knowledge do you reach understanding.'

Professor John Hyatt, 2006

CHAPTER 11

Emotional and Spiritual Care

My spiritual life is extremely important to me. I have studied with many spiritual masters and many traditions, particularly the Native American traditions, and have been fascinated by multicultural beliefs. I have been a spiritual healer for over thirty years, visiting hospices and practising from home. I am always on a journey to discover more of who I am, to connect with my heart more, and to find a more peaceful state of being. I believe that stress and unresolved emotions are one of the biggest causes of disease, and in my healing practice I work intensively to help others release the bonds of emotional stagnation and negativity that have stunted their health.

Understanding how to support the emotional and spiritual needs of those in your care, and to appreciate their importance alongside the practical aspects of care, cannot be underestimated. Spiritual care is an integral part of an older person's quality of life and can be a powerful tool to assist caring from the heart. Offering spiritual care is a quiet and largely unacknowledged two-way process that allows the frail and old to share with and minister to us, through their words and their insights. This is humbling for us and enlivening for them. It is so important to learn how to be able to give as well as receive. Offering older people the opportunity to give care themselves is like a tonic for the soul.

In 2010 the Royal College of Nursing commissioned a survey on spirituality. It revealed that members wanted:

- more education and guidance about spiritual care
- clarification about personal and professional boundaries
- support in dealing with spiritual issues

So in 2011 they published a pocket guide to *Spirituality in nursing care*. In it, they quote a definition of spiritual care from a publication by NHS Education for Scotland, 2009:

'That care which recognises and responds to the needs of the human spirit when faced with trauma, ill health or sadness and can include the need for meaning, for self worth, to express oneself, for faith support, perhaps for rites or prayer or sacrament, or simply for a sensitive listener. Spiritual care begins with encouraging human contact in compassionate relationship, and moves in whatever direction need requires.'

Spiritual needs

Spiritual care is not just about religious beliefs and practices. It is not about imposing your own beliefs and values on another, or using your position to convert. Nor is spiritual care a specialist activity or the sole responsibility of the chaplain. It is about meeting people at their deepest need. As the RCN pocket guide mentioned above says: 'Spiritual care is a fundamental part of nursing currently much neglected through ignorance and misunderstanding.'

ASCERTAINING SPIRITUAL NEEDS

You may find questions such as these from the RCN helpful when trying to unearth the spiritual needs of those you care for:

- Do you have a way of making sense of the things that happen to you?
- What sources of support/help do you look to when life is difficult?
- Would you like to see someone who can help you?
- Would you like to see someone who can help you talk or think through the impact of this illness/life event? (You don't have to be religious to talk to them.)

It is so valuable to have an understanding of the spiritual needs older people may have, in order to empathise, encourage and support these important aspects of human nature. Some of these spiritual needs may be:

- to have meaning and purpose
- to be able to rise above circumstances
- to be able to pass things on
- to receive support in times of loss
- to experience a sense of continuity in life
- to have encouragement and support for faith activities and rituals
- to maintain personal dignity and a sense of worth
- to receive unconditional love and compassion
- to express feelings

- to forgive/be forgiven
- to be loved and to love
- to be respected, not patronised
- to keep and develop a sense of humour
- to develop sensitivity and imagination
- to rejoice in remaining skills and be thankful
- to keep a balance between resting and being active
- to experience surprise, anticipation, and having something to look forward to
- to enjoy creativity, seasons, nature, simple pleasures, daily living activities
- to be listened to and to have time alone to think, nurture faith and continue learning
- to discover ways to prepare for one's own death
- to nurture a sense of hope
- to have a sense of belonging

(Adapted from Spiritual Needs of Frail Older People, © *Rosemary Hurtley)*

SUPPORTING SPIRITUAL NEEDS

A lack of meaning and hope can be a source of depression in older people, causing them to withdraw from social situations. Without positive intervention this can lead to a downward spiral of their health and wellbeing. Spirituality can be used to inform and help us to facilitate healing or recovery and should be expressed meaningfully in a care plan. As people age and cope with increasing frailty, spirituality can become increasingly important. There may be an ever-increasing need to share, to express oneself and hand down what has been learnt through the years.

How do any of the spiritual needs of older people differ from your own needs?

Some ways to help support these needs are:

- by encouraging elders to enjoy life by using their existing abilities
- by encouraging others to share their emotions, feelings, hopes and fears
- by supporting the inner values and beliefs that help people cope
- by building relationships and getting to know individuals so that you can think about how to provide a varied and interesting day
- by recognising the themes, symbols and religious cultures that are important to the people in your care
- by paying attention to your own spiritual needs; if you feel out of your depth, seek help from someone you trust or contact interfaith ministers or other support networks
- by knowing your own strengths and limitations

Be aware of when it is appropriate to refer to another source of support such as a chaplain, counsellor, family member or friend.

Tools for emotional and spiritual support

ACTIVE LISTENING

Active listening is a powerful tool to support the emotional needs of others. Having regrets, loss, unresolved difficulties or relationships can be a legitimate source of stress. Some older people may want to reflect on these and perhaps share with others who will listen to help them to resolve difficulties in their minds or to accept their situation.

ACTIVE LISTENING EXERCISE

In my workshops I ask participants to sit in pairs and take it in turns to share a powerful memory. I then ask them to repeat back to each other the memory they had been told by the other person. People are often alarmed by this, but it is an exercise to see how well we listen and how much empathy we have for the emotion of that other person. It is amazing how easy it is for us to appear to be listening while our mind wanders. But once the students experience attentive/active listening, each pair feels validated and able to reach a clearer perspective on their own memory too.

Sometimes, all we need is to be fully present in a situation. This benefits those we care for, but also releases us from outside interference which can prevent us from giving the quality of care we wish to give.

JUST BE

Spirituality is a personal and important part of an older person's journey from 'doing' to 'being'. The simplest definition of spirituality is that aspect of us that gives meaning and purpose to life. It is about being connected with creation (God, a higher power, great spirit), ourselves and our feelings, and being connected to others.

'JUST BEING' EXERCISE

I love this quote by Richard Allen: 'We work not to provide answers but friendship, to share, not to solve. We bring no one but ourselves, and that is our greatest gift.' I share the quote with groups before the following exercise.

I ask participants in my workshops to pair up, with one sitting and the other standing behind them. I tell them that for the next five minutes they will not have to do anything, just *be*, be who they are with the person in front of them. There is nothing to fix, do or say; this is an opportunity to simply *be* with another human being who is also simply going to *be*. Know that being who you are is enough. I ask the person standing behind to put their hands on the sitting person's shoulders. That will be the only physical connection. Then I ask both partners to please close their eyes and allow their feet to feel rooted to the earth.

In that five minutes of silence it is so gratifying to see a room full of people relaxed yet connected. It is a powerful exercise, and often people are in tears afterwards. Feedback from those seated has included: 'I felt honoured, in a strange way, by the person standing'; 'I felt great heat and comfort from the hands on my shoulders'; 'I felt deeply relaxed'; 'I felt supported in a way I can't explain'.

The feedback from those standing has included: 'I felt so peaceful'; 'I felt loved and loving'; 'I felt strong, grounded, energised'.

This exercise demonstrates to me that our presence, our essence, can be enough to restore peace and healing in just five minutes, without the need to perform tasks or even talk. It is so important to allow ourselves time to just be, and to connect without words allows a different and profound form of communication which can restore our spirit.

MEMORIES AS A SPIRITUAL BALM

Whatever our faith, or lack of it, in old age the human need to put things in order, forgive, be listened to, receive sanctuary, peace, acceptance, hope, understanding and support becomes important. As we reach old age we have a lifetime's experience on which to reflect, and those of us who work with older people can travel as co-explorers with those who invite us. There is a treasure chest of life experiences and stories which can be shared. Memories can access, help and nurture spiritual growth.

SHARING WISDOM

In later life, some older people have a deep need to share what they have learned and to hand down a rich vein of life experience. Provide opportunities for this sharing, and acknowledge their value by giving them a diary to write in, by videoing them or by making voice recordings. Leaving the bubble of our busy lives to enter the bubble of people's lived experience is also the essence of good quality care when looking after those with dementia. In your care of another person, consider how many ways you may be able to provide opportunities for reciprocal care. You may find yourself pleasantly on the receiving end.

GRATITUDE

You may encounter various states of depression in yourself and in those you care for; a balm for these dark times that is drug free and cost free is deep gratitude. This may sound trite, but I have seen so many times how gratitude can lighten mental states.

'Be thankful.' This is an old adage, but one that can have a profound effect on our attitude to life and to others. The 'attitude of gratitude' inspires the ability to see the world through fresh eyes, to be appreciative and to value the positive aspects of ourselves, our colleagues and those we care for rather than finding fault.

'BE THANKFUL' EXERCISE

Think of one thing you can be grateful for today. This can range from the small to the universal: a cup of tea, the flowers by the bedside, a smile, the planet. Write this down, then encourage those in your care to find one thing they can be grateful for. I like to expand this exercise by asking participants in my workshops to write a list of everything they are thankful for. Write for five minutes, then share your list with others to appreciate how these gifts can enrich our daily lives. You may want to consider keeping a 'count your blessings' journal which can be added to in the future. Or you could start a gratitude circle where staff, residents and relatives join to express and share their blessings.

IT ONLY TAKES A MINUTE

The Janki Foundation is a wonderful organisation led by its spiritual leader, Dadi Janki. I had the privilege of interviewing her for my film *The Big Adventure*. When I visited the head-quarters of her spiritual university Brahma Kumaris to film, I was told that we would have to stop for a minute every hour when a bell was rung. This, Dadi explained to me, was so that everyone had the opportunity to stop what they were doing and reconnect with themselves for just one minute of silence every hour.

From spending just one day there I could see the value of this. It may be something you wish to do for yourself: to stop the world, to regroup, re-centre yourself, particularly when feeling overwhelmed while caring for others. It only takes a minute. Try it and see.

NOURISHING THE SOUL

One of the exercises I like doing with my workshop participants is the following Janki exercise. It can positively change the
energy of the group for quite some time afterwards. If you try
it, don't limit it to staff; enjoy exploring it with the elders you
care for too. Relish these opportunities to connect and share.

APPRECIATION EXERCISE

Think of something that would be nourishing to you, something said
or done that you would really appreciate. Write down on a card what
that 'gift' could be. Write it as a positive statement, for example: 'You
are always so kind'; 'You make me laugh'; 'You cheer me up'. Allow
two or three minutes for this.

Now walk slowly around the room, holding up your card. Whenever
you meet someone, stop and greet them and exchange cards. Read
their card and take it on as a personal compliment. Move on and
exchange cards with someone else. Allow another two or three minutes, until everyone has exchanged cards.

Sit quietly with the card you have at the end, contemplating the
gift for a few moments.

Spiritual recipes

Write your own 'spiritual recipe', using the example overleaf,
then swap spiritual recipes with others. It is an engaging way to
remind yourself and others of your deeper needs, and it is a useful
way to help those you care for to open up about their own needs.

*A good measure of reflection and beauty, a sprinkling of thought-
fulness, a large tablespoon of empathetic listening and kindness.
Thoroughly mix with appreciation and understanding. Take a tea-
spoon of humour and mix with creativity and playfulness, then
thoroughly mix with love. Sprinkle with hope to garnish.*

FOOD FOR THOUGHT

Consider having a small library of books, quotations, poetry,
relaxation CDs, religious texts, self-help manuals and travel
journals that can support the emotional and spiritual needs of
yourself and others. Perhaps expand this by reading to each
other and encouraging personal reviews of each book, explaining how they helped and why.

NATURE, A GIFT THAT LIFTS!

Do not underestimate the soothing and healing power of
nature for yourself and those in your care. Consider walking
where possible in beautiful surroundings, or bringing the natural world indoors if mobility is a problem. Shells, pine cones,
flowers, bonsai trees, and CDs of waves, birdsong and other
natural sounds can all help us reconnect with the world
around us.

MUSIC FOR THE SPIRIT

Music can inspire, motivate, soothe and calm. Listen to different types of music to create an atmosphere of peace or joy or
whatever is appropriate to support the emotional needs of
those in your care. You can be a spiritual DJ and consider all
genres of music!

IDENTIFYING VALUES AS SPIRITUAL TOOLS

Mother Theresa said of her personal values: 'The three most important things in life are to be kind, to be kind, to be kind.'

Values can be described as core beliefs or principles. It is important to identify your values, as they determine what you bring to your work environment and form the basis of your actions with the older people you support. When we act in accordance with our personal values, we act from strength in a humane and harmonious fashion, with greater contentment and satisfaction in our personal and working life.

VALUES EXERCISE

Consider for yourself what values you live by and why. Try to discover the values of those you care for, as they reveal so much about a person. During times of crisis we can help remind each other to remain true to our values.

To help you identify your values, consider the list below to see which most resonate with you:

acceptance, appreciation, balance, benevolence, clarity, 'centredness', commitment, compassion, co-operation, courage, dependability, dignity, enthusiasm, forgiveness, flexibility, generosity, gratitude, honesty, hope, humour, inspiration, integrity, kindness, love, loyalty, openness, patience, peace, practicality, respect, responsibility, tolerance, trust, wisdom.

No regrets

There may be a battle within an older person as they get ready to 'pack their bags' to address regrets, and one of the

most important things you can do as a carer to the dying is
to provide opportunities for the mending of broken/troubled
relationships. Regrets at what one might have done, could
have done, should have done may surface quite dramatically
for older people when they are faced with life-threatening
illness. Gentle empathetic and emotional skills are needed to
guide them through the mire of self-recrimination, anger or
loss.

One of the most common causes of grief, which can entrap
many in a whirlpool of mourning that is so difficult to tran-
scend, is when a loved one dies without expressing their love
for you, or if you were unable to say goodbye or tell them that
you love them. My short film *No Regrets* covers this aspect in a
powerful ten-minute drama that packs an emotional punch
with an unexpected twist. This film triggers greater awareness
in professional carers of the relative's experience, an important
aspect that is all too often neglected. Absence of love or forgiveness can eat away at those left behind; that is why I am so
pleased *No Regrets* is used in end-of-life training sessions
around the world.

We all need acknowledgement and closeness, and at the end
of a person's life it will be the love they have received that they
will remember.

'Often it is not until crisis, illness . . . or suffering occurs that
the illusion (of security) is shattered . . . illness, suffering . . .
and ultimately death . . . become spiritual encounters as well
as physical and emotional experiences'

(*Quoted as being 'Ganstrom in Hitchins, 1988' in* Spirituality in nursing
care: a pocket guide *published by the Royal College of Nursing, 2011*)

IF YOU DIED . . .

In my workshops I often read out the following letter to high-light the need for expressing love when you can. It was written by Vita Sackville-West to her husband Harold Nicholson.

> My own darling Harold,
> I was thinking this morning how awful it would be if you died.
> I do often think about that, but it came over me in all of a heap when I looked out of the bathroom window and saw you in your blue coat and black hat pottering in the garden.
> It is the sudden view of a person that twists one's heart. And I often think that I've never told you how much I love you – and if you died I should reproach myself, saying 'Why did I never tell him, why did I never tell him enough?'

IF I DIED TOMORROW

I have tried to live my life without lashing out at or hurting another person, for I know that if I did so the regret would stay with me for a long time. In my workshops I ask carers in pairs to discuss what regrets they may have at their moment of death, and to explore how the honest sharing of this exercise can help them connect with and understand the elders they care for.

I use the following poem, written by an 80-year-old woman, to encourage everyone to think about the consequences of their regrets.

> *If I had my life to live over*
> If I had my life to live over again
> I'd dare to make more mistakes.

I would take fewer things seriously,
I would take more chances,
I would take more trips.

If I had my life to live over,
I would stay barefoot
Earlier in the spring
And stay that way later in the fall.
I would go to more dances,
I would ride more merry go rounds,
I would pick more daisies.
I would climb more mountains
And swim more rivers;
I would eat more ice cream and less beans.
I would perhaps have more actual troubles
But I'd have fewer imaginary ones.

Oh, I've had my moments,
And if I had to do it over again
I'd have more of them.
In fact, I'd try to have nothing else.
Just moments, one after another,
Instead of living so many years
Ahead of each day.
If I had to do it all again,
I would travel lighter next time.

DEATH, THE LAST TABOO

I have been asked many times to take workshops on spiri-
tuality and end-of-life care and was delighted to launch the
Dying Matters coalition (www.dyingmatters.org.uk) on the
BBC. This organisation has over 16,000 members and is a

wonderful hub of ideas, knowledge and support around end-of-life care. The National Council for Palliative Care, another excellent organisation and provider of resources, commissioned me to make a film for them on end-of-life care for the more marginalised parts of society including the homeless.

I have always wanted to change society's attitude to death and dying, to see if we could change the morbid aspects of death into a celebration of the transformational aspects of one's passing. I love this quote by J.M. Barrie from *Peter Pan*: 'To die must be an awfully big adventure.' And in fact *The Big Adventure* is the title of my end-of-life short film which, through poetry, anecdote, interviews and music, provides a tapestry of thoughts and experiences to explore this seemingly taboo subject. I am so pleased that *The Big Adventure* is being used by thousands of hospices, hospitals and care homes and in end-of-life conferences to inspire debate and the exploration of the totality of our existence. The film helps us to realise that, although we value the birth companion, the death companion's role is just as important. I believe that to work with the dying is challenging but sacred work, and that death shouldn't be sanitised or brushed under the carpet. Death shouldn't be something we have to shield each other from, rather it is something we should guide each other through.

There is not enough understanding of the profound effect on staff and carers that someone's passing has, and there is little provision made for discussion around this and for the expression of spiritual beliefs. I hope my film will continue to ask the questions that will start a different approach to end-of-life care, because training in this area has been woefully pushed aside in the past.

LEAVE ROOM FOR THE UNEXPLAINED

During my mother's final weeks, when I was giving her healing, she said, 'I think I should like to come back as a butterfly.' It was a beautiful sentiment that stayed with me, one I shared with the rest of my family. When Mama did pass, on the day of her cremation I was struggling terribly with the thought of her body being burnt – her wishes, but somehow I couldn't bear the thought of this desecration to her body, as I saw it through the eyes of my grief. I was worried that I would break down uncontrollably at the point of the cremation itself. But as the curtains closed around the coffin a red admiral butterfly flew down in a shaft of sunlight and landed on the curtains at the point of closure. Well, all the congregation saw this but only my family understood its true significance. My heart lifted and I didn't break down, and the butterfly flew over our heads and out of the double doors as we left the service.

I then had a red admiral butterfly in the limousine on the way to her memorial at the Actor's Church and in my railway carriage on the way home. On the first performance of my Christmas show, which I wrote and performed with all my family, the audience knew that Virginia McKenna was replacing Mama. It was 10 December and we were performing in a stately home. During the interval in our dressing area, which was a small lounge with a beamed fireplace, out of the chimney came a red admiral butterfly which circled round my script, landed on my father's hand and flew by my musicians. At the point of 'act two beginners' being called, my father opened the tiny casement window and the butterfly flew straight out. Well, we gave the best performance ever that night and at the curtain call I felt compelled to tell the audience the story of Mama and the butterfly. To my surprise and delight we had a discussion with the audience, who were keen to share many similar stories, for over an hour.

When I tell this story during my talks I make a plea for carers to allow the space for those we care for to share their experiences of the 'unexplainable', not to dismiss these other-worldly, spiritual experiences that may provide great comfort and reassurance. Allow room for the mystery of life and death without judging or correcting the experiences of others.

AND FINALLY . . .

Before my father died I was tormented with the fear that I would be unable to reach any sort of peace with his passing, for I was riddled with unexpressed rage at aspects of his behaviour that I had endured for so long without challenging him. The truth is I loved him fiercely but was frightened of him, and rarely found the courage to challenge him or stand up for myself, choosing the path of acquiescence for fear of the consequences.

But this 'unfinished business' within myself was eating away at me. I had to find some sort of resolution, restitution and for-giveness for him and myself, to allow for a 'clean' death where we both could be liberated in our separation. I prayed for a solution and realised that I needed to speak with my father about all the positive and negative aspects of our relationship, to speak my truth. I knew that I needed this witnessed too. I called upon my second mother, Virginia McKenna, to be with me. She was close to my father too and felt like a family member, so her presence would not be inappropriate.

The day of this truth telling, this unburdening – this releas-ing, if you like – I felt calm and held Dad's hands as I spoke to him gently but freely about all aspects of our relationship. I spoke for over an hour, and Dad did not interrupt as the memories flowed through me. I asked for his forgiveness, as in the moment of speaking so honestly with him I could feel my forgiveness of him too. I thanked him for creating me, and I thanked him for the challenges he gave me. I told him that his life had enriched me, and that I would miss him, but now without my rage or anger I could let him go, sure in my belief that I would see him once more.

I washed my father's feet and combed his hair and honoured him in a way that felt right for me and him. It was a profound life-changing experience and I could feel the healing and the peace between us. I share this story at my conferences because so often the opportunity to restore and heal a relationship is left too late, as one grieves for the loss of a loved one. I want to share another way of easing the transition for those who pass and those who are left behind.

Remember even at the end of life to provide plenty of opportunities for older people to continue to grow emotionally and spiritually. The poet John Donne suggests we all need to find our place within the human family and that 'no man is an island', stressing the importance of developing relationships and connecting with ourselves and others.

My CD of songs for the dying, *I Am Near You*, is there to act as a comforting presence to someone who may be dying alone as staff and family cannot be there all the time. My unaccompanied voice singing adult lullabies and gentle songs is used in hospices and care homes to help ease the transition from this life into the Big Adventure.

Oliver Sachs wrote: 'However great the organic damage, there remains the undiminished responsibility of reintegration by art, by communion, by touching the spirit.' And I hope that this chapter has touched your spirit and will help you find ways to support the emotional and spiritual needs of yourself and others.

'Do more than belong: participate. Do more than **care**: help. Do more than believe: practise. Do more than be fair: be kind. Do more than forgive: forget. Do more than dream: work.'

William Arthur Ward

BIBLIOGRAPHY AND FURTHER READING

I recommend the following publications if you would like to learn more about caring from the heart.

Allen R *(2008) Wholeness in the Fourth Age: Journeying into Freedom, the Spiritual Care of Older People*

Allan H, Smith P *(2005) The Introduction of Modern Matrons and the Relevance of Emotional Labour to Understanding their Roles: Developing Personal Authority in Clinical Leadership* (pp 20-32), International Journal of Work, Organisation and Emotion, Vol 1, No 1, ed: Sue Simpson and Steve Smith

Alcoe J *(2008) Lifting Your Spirits: Seven Tools for Coping with Illness*, Janki Foundation

Bonner C *(2005) Reducing Stress-Related Behaviours in People with Dementia*, Jessica Kingsley, London

Briner R *(2005) What can Research into Emotion at Work Tell us About Researching Wellbeing at Work?* (pp 67-73), International Journal of Work Organisation and Emotion, Vol 1, No 1

British Heart Foundation *(2005) Moving More Often Programme*, BHF

Burton-Jones J, Hurtley R *(2008) Find the Right Care Home*, Age Concern England

Castledine G *(2008) The Use of Language in Nursing Care*, British Journal of Nursing (p. 615), May 2008

Covey S *(2004) Seven Effective Habits of Highly Effective People*, Franklin Covey, Free Press

Craig C, Mountain G *(2008) Lifestyle Matters*, Speechmark, Oxon

Department of Health *(2006) The Dignity Challenge*, SCIE

Duff P, Hurtley R *(2008) The Resident-Centred Care Home StandardTM* (RCC HS), User's Guide

Eden Conference, Birmingham 2006

Farmer S *(2005) The Relationships of Emotional Intelligence to Burnout and Job Satisfaction Among Nurses in Early Nursing*, (practice paper presented at first International Conference on Working with Emotions: Organisations, Occupations and Self)

Fineman S *(2005) Appreciating Emotion at Work: Paradigm Tensions* (pp 4-14), International Journal of Work Organisation and Emotion, Vol.1, No 1, ed: Sue Simpson and Steve Smith

Foote C, Stanner C *(2005) Integrating Care for Older People*, Jessica Kingsley, London

Friedan B *(1993) The Fountain of Age*, Jonathan Cape, London

Feil M *(2003) Validation; The Feil Method*, 2nd edition, Edward Feil Productions, Cleveland

Gibson *(1999) Can we Risk Person-Centred Communication?* Journal of Dementia Care, 1(5) (pp 20-24).

Goodwin P, Page T *(2008) From Hippos to Gazelles – How Leaders Create Leaders*, Kingham Press

Harrison A, Simpson R *(2005) Emotions in the Organisation*, (p. 87-102), International Journal of Work Organisation and Emotion, Vol 1, No 1, ed: Sue Simpson and Steve Smith

Help the Aged *(2006) My Home Life*, Help the Aged

Hurtley C *(2006) Coping with Stress and Burnout* (amended by R Hurtley 2009, handout)

Hurtley R, Wenborn J *(2005) The Successful Activity Co-ordinator,* Age Concern Books

James O *(2009) Contented Dementia,* Vermilion, London

Janki Foundation *(2004) Values in Healthcare,* Janki Foundation

Jewell A (ed) *(1998) Spirituality and Ageing,* Jessica Kingsley, London

Kitwood T *(1997) Dementia Reconsidered: the Person Comes First* (p 26), UK Buckingham Open University Press

Loehr R, Scwartz T *(2005) The Power of Full Engagement: How to be an Even Better Manager*

Macky H, Nancarrow S (eds) *(2008) Enabling Independence,* Blackwell Publishing

MacKinlay E *(2006) Spiritual Growth and Care in the Fourth Age of Life,* Jessica Kingsley, London

Martin M *(2009) Boredom as an Important Area for Inquiry for Occupational Therapists,* British Journal of Occupational Therapy, 72, (1), January 2009

May H, Perrin T *(2000) Wellbeing in Dementia,* Churchill Livingstone

Miall A, Milsted D *(2008) Xenophobes Guide to the English,* Oval Books

Miesen BML *(2004) The Psychology of Dementia: Awareness and Intangible Loss* (taken from **Jones GMM, Miesen (eds)** *Care-Giving Dementia: Research and Applications,* Volume 4, London, Routledge, (pp 183–213)).

NAPA *(2002) Certificate in Providing Therapeutic Activities for Older People,* City & Guilds, Trainer's Manual, NAPA

Network Training *(2005) Provision of Activities for Older People in Care Settings,* Tribal

Nolan et al *(2001),* **Nolan et al** *(2006) Quality in Ageing-Policy Practice Research,* Sept 2006, Pavilion Journals, Brighton

Nolan M, Lundh U, Grant G, Keady J *(2003) Partnerships in Family Care*, Open University Press, Maidenhead

Nightingale F *(1860) Notes on Nursing: What it is, and What it is Not*, Copyright 1969, Dover Publications Inc, NY

Owen T, The National Care Home Research and Development Forum (eds) *(2006) My Home Life: Quality in Life in Care Homes*, Help the Aged, London

Perrin T (ed) *(2004) The New Culture of Therapeutic Activity*, Speechmark, Oxon

Pool J *(2008) The Pool Activity Level (PAL) Instrument*, Jessica Kingsley, London

Ross-Smith, Chesterman, Peters M *(2005) Watch Out, Here Comes Feeling! Women Executives and Emotion Work*, (p. 48–66), International Journal of Work Organisation and Emotion, Vol 1, No 1

Sheard D *(2007) Enabling*, The Alzheimer's Society

Simpson R, Smith S *(2005) International Journal of Work Organisation and Emotion*, (Introduction pp 1–4), Vol 1, No 1

Smith P *(1992) The Emotional Labour of Nursing: How Nurses Care*, Palgrave Macmillan, Basingstoke

Smith P *(2008) Compassion and Smiles: What's the Evidence?* Journal of Research in Nursing, Sage, Vol 13(5) (pp 367–370)

Stephen Sonsino (website 2005)

Waddington K *(2005) Behind Closed Doors – The Role of Gossip in the Emotional Labour of Nursing Work* (pp 35–45), International Journal of Work Organisation and Emotion, Vol 1, No 1, ed: Sue Simpson and Steve Smith

Woods R T *(2001) Discovering the Person with Alzheimer's Disease: Cognitive, Emotional, Behavioural Aspects*, (p. 7–16), Ageing and Mental Health, 5 (1)

ACKNOWLEDGEMENTS

I would like to thank my mother and father and all of my family, particularly my son Ben for his encouragement and support. I would like to acknowledge the work of those who have inspired me in my work: Dr Bill Thomas, Dr Patch Adams, Rosemary Hurtley, Cathe Gaskill and David Sheard. I thank Ernest Hecht and Seouvenir Press for inviting me to write this book and Alison Pressley for editing it.

I would like to thank all those who have walked with me on this journey of caring from the heart, both seen and unseen, and for the continual process of learning how to give and receive love. Thank you, thank you thank you.

AFTERWORD

The Heart of Care for Ourselves

Remembering and Embracing Who We Are

Our resistance to the ageing process can hold us in a place of stagnation and regret. To free ourselves from the constraints of the perceived social stigma of ageing or being 'past it', we have to change our appreciation of ourselves to someone whose life is an amazing accumulation of lived experiences and emotions. We will then understand that the deepest challenges we have experienced have provided us with our greatest learning, and that as we age we have the opportunity to reflect on these lessons learned and become grateful and gently accepting.

But it can happen that parts of us are trapped in emotional pain, unwilling to move or grow, haunted by memories, frozen in time – as experienced by those with dementia. How do we integrate all those aspects of ourselves that may have splintered off due to trauma, shock, hurt, anger and resentment? We need to have the courage, determination and patience to listen to the part of us that is hurting so badly it affects our attitude to ourselves and others – that feeling when we sense we have lost who we are and react in a way that feels alien to us. Until recently I had completely ignored the little girl in me that had been frightened and mistrusting of what love was, and I was shocked at the realisation that I had trapped part of myself in a very lonely place. Through taking the time to sit with myself, to write a letter to my former younger self and to listen to her confusion, alienation, anger and mistrust – as painful as many of the memories and realisations were – a shift occurred that allowed me to move forward, with that aspect of myself no longer ignored or shut away but embraced and welcomed and able to grow with me.

We may often be compassionate with others, but with ourselves it can be a very different story. We must learn to be tender with ourselves, to see our complexity but also our simplicity. We all want to feel loved but rarely take the time to acknowledge the parts of ourselves that feel unworthy of being loved. We should soothe, forgive and comfort the deepest wounds we have, for the wounded parts of us will try to grab our attention in more and more persistent ways in later years.

Like a mother with a child, we can sit with that part of us that is hurting and say:

> I remember you, remembering me;
> remembering you I will not forget you,
> I will never abandon you.
> I forgive you.

These words provide the space for healing and for reintegration to take place over time. They give us the opportunity to heal ourselves; to allow all parts of ourselves to grow together restored and whole; to experience the heart of care for ourselves, which is one of our greatest gifts.